IMAGES FOR THE BOARDS:
A COMPREHENSIVE IMAGE-BASED REVIEW

USMLE Images for the Boards:

A Comprehensive Image-Based Review

Amber S. Tully, MD

Associate Staff, Department of Family Medicine, Cleveland Clinic, Cleveland, Ohio

James S. Studdiford, MD, FACP

Associate Professor, Department of Family and Community Medicine, Jefferson Medical College, Thomas Jefferson University, Philadelphia, Pennsylvania

1600 John F. Kennedy Blvd.
Ste 1800
Philadelphia, PA 19103-2899

USMLE IMAGES FOR THE BOARDS:
A COMPREHENSIVE IMAGE-BASED REVIEW   ISBN: 978-1-4557-0903-8

Notices

Knowledge and best practice in this field are constantly changing. As new research and experience broaden our understanding, changes in research methods, professional practices, or medical treatment may become necessary.

Practitioners and researchers must always rely on their own experience and knowledge in evaluating and using any information, methods, compounds, or experiments described herein. In using such information or methods they should be mindful of their own safety and the safety of others, including parties for whom they have a professional responsibility.

With respect to any drug or pharmaceutical products identified, readers are advised to check the most current information provided (i) on procedures featured or (ii) by the manufacturer of each product to be administered, to verify the recommended dose or formula, the method and duration of administration, and contraindications. It is the responsibility of practitioners, relying on their own experience and knowledge of their patients, to make diagnoses, to determine dosages and the best treatment for each individual patient, and to take all appropriate safety precautions.

To the fullest extent of the law, neither the Publisher nor the authors, contributors, or editors, assume any liability for any injury and/or damage to persons or property as a matter of products liability, negligence or otherwise, or from any use or operation of any methods, products, instructions, or ideas contained in the material herein.

International Standard Book Number
978-1-4557-0903-8

Library of Congress Cataloging-in-Publication Data
Tully, Amber.
    USMLE images for the boards : an image based review / Amber Tully, James S. Studdiford.
       p. ; cm.
    Includes bibliographical references and index.
    ISBN 978-1-4557-0903-8 (pbk. : alk. paper)
    I. Studdiford, James S. II. Title.
    [DNLM: 1. Clinical Medicine–Examination Questions. WB 18.2]
    LC classification not assigned
    616.0076–dc23
                              2012001897

Content Strategy Director: Madelene Hyde
Senior Content Strategist: James Merritt
Senior Content Coordinator: Margaret Nelson
Publishing Services Manager: Patricia Tannian/Hemamalini Rajendrababu
Senior Project Manager: Sarah Wunderly
Project Manager: Prathibha Mehta
Senior Book Designer: Louis Forgione

Printed in China

Last digit is the print number: 9 8 7 6 5 4 3 2 1

Dedication

The "boards" book is dedicated to our students and residents, past, present, and future, who serve as our greatest teachers.

About the Authors

Amber Stonehouse Tully, MD, is Associate Staff in the Department of Family Medicine at the Cleveland Clinic. She has a special interest in dermatology, plastic surgery, physical diagnosis, and clinical images. While a medical student she co-developed a medical imaging database, Jefferson Clinical Images (JCI), which currently holds over 1200 images, boards review questions, clinical cases, and lectures. Dr. Tully enjoys medical writing and has published several papers in peer-reviewed journals. She and Dr. Studdiford created Top Doc, a medical quiz iPhone app released in 2010. Dr. Tully has received several leadership awards, including the Family Medicine Education Consortium Emerging Leader Award, AAFP/Bristol Myers Squibb Award for Excellence in Graduate Medical Education, the William Potter Memorial Prize in Clinical Medicine, the Arthur Krieger Memorial Prize in Family Medicine, the Drs. Ronald R. and Henry Pohl Prize for Professionalism, and the J. Savacool Prize in Medical Ethics.

James S. Studdiford, MD, FACP, is an Associate Professor of Family and Community Medicine at Jefferson Medical College of Thomas Jefferson University. He has a special interest in medical photography; he founded and developed a medical imaging database, Jefferson Clinical Images (JCI), in conjunction with Academic Information Services and Research of Scott Memorial library at Thomas Jefferson University. The JCI database includes write-ups for each image and exceeds 1000 entries. Doctor Studdiford also has an active interest in medical student education. He has received several awards for teaching, including Senior Class Portrait, Humanism in Medicine Award, and The Lindback Award for Distinguished Teaching in a Clinical Science. He has also delivered The Oath of Hippocrates for the graduating senior class of Jefferson Medical College on several occasions.

Contributors and Consultants

SENIOR CONTRIBUTORS

Cindy Finden, MD
Assistant Clinical Professor of Radiology, Department of Radiology, Thomas Jefferson University Hospital, Philadelphia, Pennsylvania

Steven G. Finden, MD, DDS
Assistant Professor of Radiology, Division of Neuroradiology/ ENT, Thomas Jefferson University Hospital, Philadelphia, Pennsylvania

Gregary D. Marhefka, MD, FACC
Assistant Professor of Medicine, Department of Internal Medicine, Division of Cardiology, Jefferson Heart Institute, Philadelphia, Pennsylvania

Jeffrey Mathews, MD
Resident, Department of Radiology, Thomas Jefferson University Hospital, Philadelphia, Pennsylvania

Kathryn P. Trayes, MD
Assistant Professor, Department of Family and Community Medicine, Jefferson Medical College, Thomas Jefferson University, Philadelphia, Pennsylvania

Contributors

Abel Morris Bumgarner, MD
Jefferson Medical College, Thomas Jefferson University, Philadelphia, Pennsylvania

Jessica Hamilton, MD, MPH
Kaiser Permanente East Bay OB/GYN Residency Program, Oakland, California

Joseph Mega, MD, MPH
Department of Family Medicine, Contra Costa Regional Medical Center, Martinez, California

Jolion McGreevy, MD, MBE, MPH
Resident, Department of Emergency Medicine, Boston Medical Center, Boston, Massachusetts

Samantha A. Smith, MD
Resident, Department of Family Medicine, York Hospital, York, Pennsylvania

SENIOR CONSULTANTS

Joshua H. Barash, MD
Assistant Professor, Department of Family and Community Medicine, Jefferson Medical College, Thomas Jefferson University, Philadelphia, Pennsylvania

Geoffrey D. Mills, MD, PhD
Assistant Professor, Department of Family and Community Medicine and Department of Physiology, Assistant Residency Program Director, Jefferson Medical College, Thomas Jefferson University, Philadelphia, Pennsylvania

Louis R. Petrone, MD
Clinical Assistant Professor, Department of Family and Community Medicine, Jefferson Medical College, Thomas Jefferson University, Philadelphia, Pennsylvania

George Valko, MD
Gustave and Valla Amsterdam Professor of Family and Community Medicine, Vice-Chair for Clinical Programs, Department of Family and Community Medicine, Jefferson Medical College, Thomas Jefferson University, Philadelphia, Pennsylvania

Consultants

Armonde Baghdanian, MD
Jefferson Medical College, Thomas Jefferson University, Philadelphia, Pennsylvania

Arthur Baghdanian, MD
Jefferson Medical College, Thomas Jefferson University, Philadelphia, Pennsylvania

Victor A. Diaz, Jr., MD
Assistant Professor, Assistant Medical Director, Director, Quality Improvement, Jefferson Family Medicine Associates, Philadelphia, Pennsylvania

Alison Grant, MD
Resident, Crozer-Keystone Family Medicine, Springfield, Pennsylvania

Mohit Gupta, MD
Jefferson Medical College, Thomas Jefferson University, Philadelphia, Pennsylvania

Anne Nason Hackman, MD
Instructor, Department of Family and Community Medicine, Thomas Jefferson University Hospital, Philadelphia, Pennsylvania

Thomas M. Kennedy, MD
Jefferson Medical College, Thomas Jefferson University, Philadelphia, Pennsylvania

Daila Pravs, MD
Instructor, Department of Family and Community Medicine, Jefferson Medical College, Thomas Jefferson University, Philadelphia, Pennsylvania

Trisha Schimek, MD, MSPH
Jefferson Medical College, Thomas Jefferson University, Philadelphia, Pennsylvania

Kevin Charles Scott, MD
Instructor and Primary Care Research Fellow, Department of Family and Community Medicine, Jefferson Medical College, Thomas Jefferson University, Philadelphia, Pennsylvania

Priya Sharma
Third Year Medical Student, Jefferson Medical College, Thomas Jefferson University, Philadelphia, Pennsylvania

Contents

Introduction

Each chapter of medical education is marked by examinations—course exams, shelf exams, board exams, practical exams, licensing exams—all of which strive to recreate the patient and the disease. A large emphasis in medical education is placed on making these examinations more like real patient encounters. The majority of board examinations are compiled of traditional multiple choice questions, but more images are being used in questions to better simulate authentic clinical presentations. In teaching and preparing medical students and residents for board examinations, we have repeatedly heard complaints about limited exposure to clinical, radiographic, and electrocardiographic images. There is a paucity of board review materials that highlight images likely to be seen in increasing quantity on board examinations. Our goal for this book is to solve that problem.

The material from this book has been drawn from medical images, radiographic findings, and electrocardiograms compiled at Thomas Jefferson University. We have had an amazing group of cardiologists, radiologists, and primary care physicians aid us in collecting these images, creating challenging board-style review questions and including high-yield explanations of each disease entity outlined. Each case presented in this book is a "classic" finding likely to be seen on board examinations. The goal of the "boards" book is to provide a solid study tool to be used by students preparing for each USMLE examination and primary care board examinations.

We would like to acknowledge the editorial staff at Elsevier, especially Nicole Dicicco and Margaret Nelson, who have worked patiently with us and supported us in the creation of this book. We sincerely hope that these carefully selected images and cases provide the reader with a stimulating and challenging review.

Amber Stonehouse Tully, MD
James S. Studdiford, MD, FACP

Section I
BOARD IMAGES

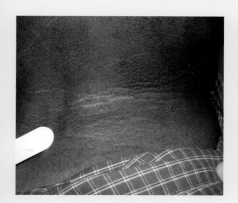 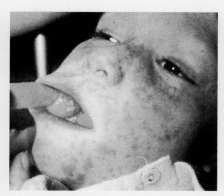 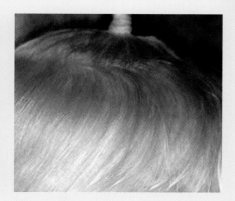

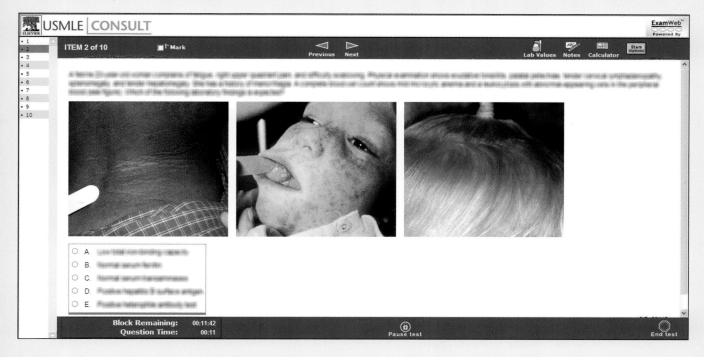

- A.
- B.
- C.
- D.
- E.

✎ *Notes*

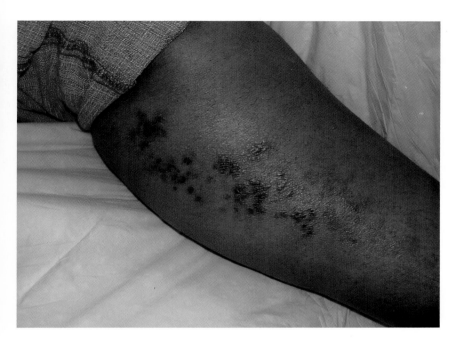

1. A 45-year-old woman presents to clinic with a new pruritic rash on the flexor surface of her left forearm. Her medical history is significant for Wilson disease, and she was recently started on penicillamine, a copper-chelator. On exam she has Kayser-Fleischer rings in both eyes and purple, polyangular papules on her left forearm. On closer inspection, fine white streaks cover the surface of the papules. A clinical diagnosis of lichen planus is made. Penicillamine is discontinued. What is the best treatment option at this time?

A. Oral steroids
B. Oral antihistamine
C. Topical steroids
D. Azathioprine
E. B and C only

2. A 36-year-old man presents to the clinic with a pruritic rash on his scalp, neck, and back. His social history is significant for intravenous (IV) drug use. On exam, violaceous, polygonal papules are noted in clusters on the scalp, neck, and back. White striae are noted on the lesional surfaces. On buccal mucosa there are tender, dendritic, lacy, white lesions bilaterally. Which of the following is/are true regarding his diagnosis?

A. Can be associated with chronic HCV
B. Disease is treated with oral steroids
C. The course can be chronic
D. Disease is treated with topical steroids
E. All of the above

1. **The answer is E: B and C only.** This patient has lichen planus (LP) as a cutaneous inflammatory reaction to penicillamine. Clinical identifiers for LP include the Four Ps (purple, polygonal, pruritic, papules), as well as Wickham striae, the fine white lines covering the papules. Other drug exposures that have been linked with LP include gold, chloroquine, and methyldopa. This is a local rash, so the best initial treatment would be topical steroid and oral antihistamine for relief from itching (**E**). Oral steroids and more potent immune modulators (azathioprine, cyclosporine) should be used with more generalized, systemic LP.

2. **The answer is E: All of the above.** This patient has oral and cutaneous lichen planus (LP) most likely related to chronic HCV status. Biopsies on dermal and oral lesions reveal mononuclear cells at the dermoepidermal junction and a T cell–mediated cytotoxic reaction against keratinocytes. HCV is thought to trigger LP via dermal and mucous membrane replication. LP usually affects flexor surfaces such as the wrists, pretibial shafts, scalp, trunk, and glans penis, and may also involve the buccal mucosa, tongue, and lips. This patient has local cutaneous lesions that could be treated with topical steroids. However, due to his buccal mucosa LP he should be started on a short course of oral prednisone (**E**). Antihistamines should also be used to treat pruritis. The course of LP is largely unpredictable, ranging from spontaneous remission to chronic eruption.

Lichen Planus

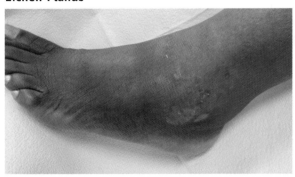

Lichen planus is a common, distinct inflammatory disorder that affects the skin, mucous membranes, nails, and hair. Lesions appear as symmetric, grouped, erythematous to violaceous, flat-topped, polygonal papules. Close inspection of the lesions with a hand lens and after application of mineral oil will reveal fine white lines (Wickham striae). Etiology of the dermatosis is diverse and includes drugs, metals, and infections (especially hepatitis C), which result in alterations of cell-mediated immunity. Women are affected more often than men, and the typical age of onset is between 30 and 60. Trauma may cause the Koebner phenomenon and linear arrangements. Treatment is with topical and systemic corticosteroids or cyclosporine.

- Four Ps: purple, polygonal, pruritic, papules
- Cutaneous lesions: distributed typically on flexural aspects of arms and legs but may become generalized; symptom is pruritis
- Oral lesions: milky-white reticulated papules, which may become erosive or ulcerate; symptom is pain

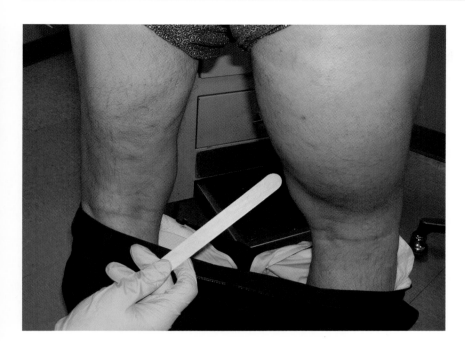

3. A 47-year-old man presents with a painless enlarging mass on the back of his right upper leg. He has no tenderness over the area, and the mass is firm on palpation. A biopsy reveals a leiomyosarcoma. All of the following are true except:

A. This tumor grows by direct local extension.
B. This tumor is derived from mature fat cells.
C. This tumor is derived from embryonic mesoderm.
D. Treatment options are guided by biopsy results.
E. The main prognostic factors are tumor grade and tumor size.

3. **The answer is B: This tumor is derived from mature fat cells.** Tumors or mature fat cells (**B**) are seen in benign lipomas rather than sarcomas. This man has a leiomyosarcoma, which is a malignant cancer derived from embryonic mesoderm (**C**). This tumor grows by direct local extension (**A**). Treatment options are guided by biopsy results (**D**) and the main prognostic factors are tumor grade and tumor size (**E**). Thus all of the above are true of sarcomas except (**B**).

Sarcoma

A *sarcoma* is a malignant neoplasm that arises from mesenchymal embryonic cells and affects connective tissue cells such as bone, cartilage, muscles, blood vessels, or fat cells. Sarcomas can be divided into two groups: those derived from bone and those derived from soft tissue. These tumors are often highly aggressive, and biopsy is required for identification of cancer cells and to guide treatment. Imaging such as ultrasound, computed tomography (CT), or magnetic resonance imaging (MRI) may be useful before biopsy is performed. Treatment options include surgical excision, radiation, and chemotherapy. In adults the most common histopathologic subtypes are liposarcoma and leiomyosarcoma, and the most common sites of origin are the thigh, buttock, and groin. In children, small cell sarcomas (e.g., Ewing sarcoma, embryonal rhabdomyosarcoma, and primitive neuroectodermal tumor) are most common.

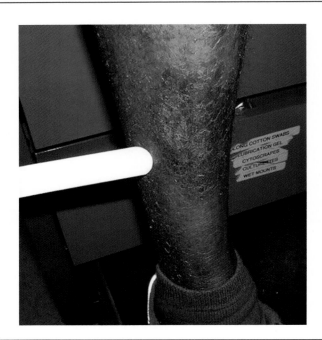

Kaposi Sarcoma

Kaposi sarcoma (KS) is the only sarcoma that is associated with a virus.

■ Grows by direct local extension

■ Soft tissue sarcoma that often presents as painless, enlarging mass
■ Main prognostic factors are grade and tumor size.
■ Radiation exposure is a risk factor for soft tissue sarcomas.

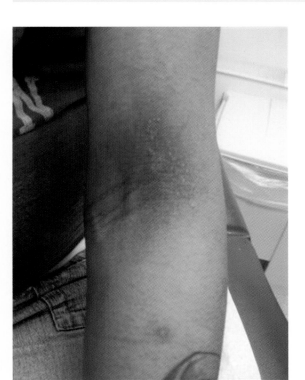

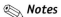
Notes

4. A 33-year-old man comes to the clinic in the winter with complaints of dry, itchy skin on his forearms (shown above) and eyelids, as well as in the creases of his elbows and knees. His past medical history is significant for mild, persistent asthma and seasonal allergies. He says that since childhood this problem has occurred annually in winter, when his asthma is also worse than usual. During the visit he is visibly uncomfortable and often scratches his arms. Which of the following should be considered when using a topical corticosteroid to treat this condition?

A. Topical corticosteroids are contraindicated in the setting of secondary staphylococcal infection.
B. Skin bleaching can occur with chronic use.
C. Application near the eye increases risk for ocular side effects.
D. Application over a large surface area can cause systemic corticosteroid effects.
E. All of the above

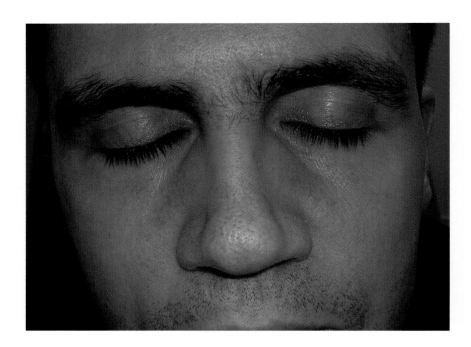

5. A 27-year-old man complains of an itchy rash on his face. The rash appeared just after he returned from a day at the beach. He recently bought a new sunscreen that he first used two weeks ago. He used the same sunscreen on his face during his most recent trip to the beach. He has had similar rashes throughout his life. He has a history of hay fever and mild asthma. Other than discontinuing use of the sunscreen, which of the following preventive measures should be recommended?

A. Limit the number of showers per day
B. Use a drying soap
C. Take hot baths
D. Apply topical corticosteroid daily
E. Apply antibacterial ointment daily

4. **The answer is E: All of the above.** This patient has atopic dermatitis (eczema). The classic triad of atopic disease includes asthma, allergic rhinitis, and atopic dermatitis. Topical corticosteroids are used to treat subacute, scaly lesions or chronic, dry, lichenified lesions of atopic dermatitis. They must, however, be used with caution for all of the reasons listed above (**E**). Patients with eczema are at an increased risk of developing a secondary infection, commonly due to staphylococcus, which is a contraindication to topical corticosteroids. Chronic use of topical corticosteroids may cause skin bleaching, and the risk of systemic side effects increases with application over a large surface area or in smaller individuals. Use on the eyelids is not recommended due to the risk of developing cataracts or glaucoma.

5. **The answer is A: Limit the number of showers per day.** Prevention of atopic dermatitis (eczema) includes avoidance of known triggers. In this case, sunscreen triggered the most recent reaction; however, other agents may have been associated with the patient's past rashes. Patients should not take hot baths (**C**) or multiple showers per day (**A**), and they should avoid drying soaps (**B**). Topical steroids can be used for subacute and chronic reactions but not as a preventive measure (**D**). Steroids should be used with caution on the face. Eczema puts patients at increased risk of secondary bacterial infection, but prophylaxis with a topical antibacterial ointment is typically not indicated (**E**).

Atopic Dermatitis (Eczema)

Atopic dermatitis is an inflammatory skin disease. It stems from a mixture of genetic susceptibility, defects in the innate immune system, and increased immunologic responses to allergens. Most patients show signs of skin disease before age 5. Lesions have a different appearance based on the duration (acute versus subacute versus chronic) and the age of the patient. Young patients often have a rash on the face and extensor surfaces, while adults have a rash on the flexural surfaces of the elbows and knees.

- Commonly associated with a personal and family history of asthma and allergic rhinitis (atopic triad)
- Decreased skin barrier protection leads to an increased risk of secondary bacterial infection.
- Preventive treatment includes moisturizers and avoidance of known triggers.
- Subacute or chronic lesions are treated with topical corticosteroids.

Notes _____

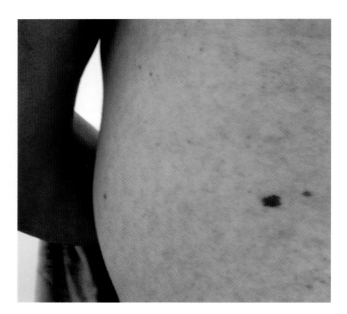

6. A 20-year-old man presents with a 0.5-cm flat nonpalpable hyperpigmented lesion on his trunk. How would you classify his primary skin lesion?

    A. Macule
    B. Patch
    C. Plaque
    D. Papule
    E. Lichenification

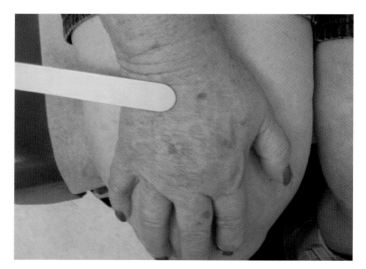

7. A 75-year-old woman presents with several lesions on the dorsal surface of both of her hands. These hyperpigmented lesions are flat and nonpalpable, have distinct borders, and range from 0.1 to 0.8 cm in size. Which of the following best classifies this primary skin lesion?

    A. Patch
    B. Plaque
    C. Papule
    D. Macule
    E. Nodule

6. **The answer is A: Macule.** This patient has a macule (**A**) because it is a flat lesion less than 10 mm in diameter. A patch (**B**) is a larger nonpalpable lesion greater than 10 mm. Plaques (**C**) are elevated palpable lesions greater than 1 cm. Papules (**D**) are palpable lesions less than 5 mm. Lichenification (**E**) is a secondary skin lesion characterized by epidermal thickening. Visible and palpable skin thickening is often present with accentuated skin markings.

7. **The answer is D: Macule.** This patient has several macules (**D**) on the dorsal surface of her hands, likely representing benign lesions called solar lentigines.

The term *macule* is used to classify any flat lesion of less than 10 mm in diameter that is even with the surface of surrounding skin and differs in color from the surrounding skin or mucous membrane. Macules may be hyperpigmented, hypopigmented, or depigmented. Patches (**A**) are larger, flat nonpalpable lesions measuring greater than 10 mm in size. Plaques (**B**) are elevated palpable lesions greater than 10 mm. Papules (**C**) are palpable lesions less than 5 mm. A nodule (**E**) is a solid, round, or ellipsoidal palpable lesion with a diameter larger than 5 mm. Nodules are differentiated from papules and plaques by depth of involvement and/or substantive palpability.

Macule

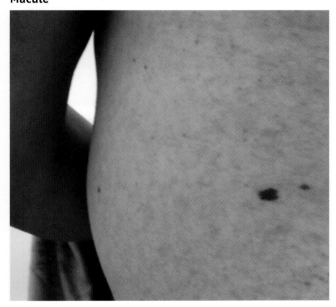

A *macule* is a primary skin lesion defined by a nonpalpable change in surface color without elevation or depression that is generally less than 10 mm in size.

- Flat, nonpalpable, less than 10 mm
- Primary skin lesion
- Examples include vitiligo, tinea versicolor, café au lait spots, mongolian spots, freckles.

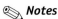 *Notes*

_____

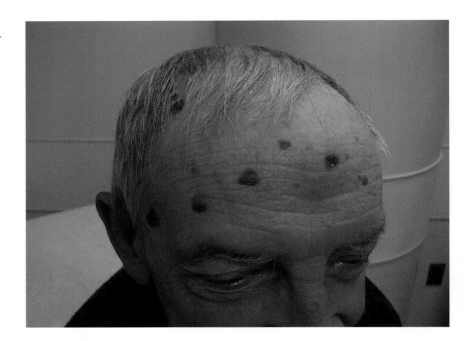

8. A 69-year-old man presents with several exophytic, brown papules and plaques that appear as though they could be scraped off. What typical finding would you expect to see on histology?

A. Islands of proliferating epithelium resembling the basal layer of the epidermis

B. Hyperplasia of benign, basaloid epidermal cells with horn pseudocysts

C. Focal increase in melanocytes

D. Intraepidermal atypia over a sun-damaged dermis

E. Intraepidermal atypical keratinocytes with penetration of the basement membrane

9. A 74-year-old man comes to you, his new primary care physician, after being urged by his granddaughter to get some spots on his back looked at. Physical exam demonstrates numerous "stuck-on," waxy, verrucous papules and plaques of various sizes and colors. Which of the following is correct regarding this man's condition?

A. These growths originate in keratinocytes.

B. Similar to warts, these lesions are viral in origin.

C. These lesions, if left untreated, may progress to melanoma.

D. Histologic examination would demonstrate a focal increase in melanocytes.

E. These growths could have been avoided if adequate preventive measures had been taken.

8. **The answer is B: Hyperplasia of benign, basaloid epidermal cells with horn pseudocysts.** These warty, brown lesions with a "stuck-on" appearance are seborrheic keratoses. Biopsy would show hyperplasia of benign, basaloid epidermal cells with horn pseudocysts (**B**). Horn pseudocysts are virtually pathognomonic. Islands of proliferating epithelium resembling the basal layer of the epidermis (**A**) is the histologic finding in basal cell carcinoma. A focal increase in melanocytes (**C**) is seen in lentigo. Intraepidermal atypia over a sun-damaged dermis (**D**) is seen in actinic keratosis. Intraepidermal atypical keratinocytes with penetration of the basement membrane (**E**) is indicative of squamous cell carcinoma.

9. **The answer is A: These growths originate in keratinocytes.** These warty brown lesions are seborrheic keratoses and originate in keratinocytes, hence the name (**A**). While these lesions are often referred to as *seborrheic warts*, there is not a viral association (**B**). These lesions are benign in nature and do not commonly progress to melanoma (**C**). A focal increase in melanocytes is seen in lentigo (**D**). While preventive measures such as sunscreen use and protective clothing are useful to prevent malignant skin lesions, seborrheic keratoses, commonly referred to as *age barnacles,* are simply a product of aging.

Seborrheic Keratosis

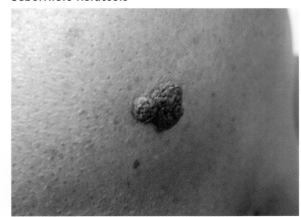

Seborrheic keratoses are raised 3- to 20-mm lesions with a stuck-on appearance. They can be flat or raised and typically have a velvety or warty surface. Although the lesions are often hyperpigmented, they range in color from light tan to black. These benign epidermal growths are a result of proliferation of immature keratinocytes. They tend to develop after age 50. Atypical lesions can be biopsied to rule out cancer. Shave biopsy reveals horn cysts which are virtually pathognomonic. Usually no treatment is necessary, but surgical excision is an option for cosmetic reasons.

- Increased incidence with increasing age
- Common benign skin growth
- Biopsy shows horn cysts
- No treatment necessary

✎ *Notes*

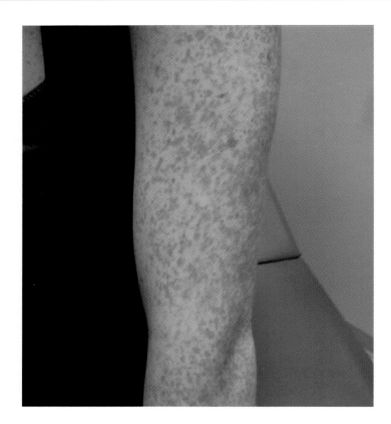

10. On a routine well-child exam of an 8-year-old girl, the patient's mother raises concern for her daughter's susceptibility to skin cancer due to the patient's fair complexion with many freckles on her face and extremities. The patient's mother notes that her daughter's skin burns easily when out in the sun. Most of the family is unable to tan with sun exposure. Her family history is significant for a maternal grandmother with basal cell carcinoma and paternal aunt with melanoma. On exam the patient is a healthy, fair-complexioned girl with light blue irides and areas of dense ephelides (freckles) on her face, shoulders, arms, and legs. You counsel the patient and her mother of her risk of skin cancer. Which of the following provide(s) effective prevention for skin cancer in this patient?

A. Avoid excessive sun and ultraviolet (UV) light exposure.
B. Use titanium dioxide and zinc oxide sunscreens.
C. Use hydroquinone to bleach freckles.
D. Use skin-covering clothing and hats.
E. All of the above
F. Only A, B, and D

10. **The answer is F: Only A, B, and D.** This patient exhibits the phenotype of those with the highest lifetime risk of skin cancer (melanoma, basal cell carcinoma, squamous cell carcinoma): fair skin with an abundance of freckles, light irides usually with blond or red hair, unable to tan, and easily sunburned. Exposure to ultraviolet A (UVA) and ultraviolet B (UVB) light poses a higher risk in these individuals. Frequent UV light exposure and blistering childhood sunburns put these individuals at higher risk for melanoma. Chronic UV light exposure correlates more with a higher risk of basal cell carcinoma and squamous cell carcinoma. Paramount to skin cancer prevention is avoiding and blocking exposure to UVA and UVB light (**F**). Hydroquinone has been shown to bleach freckles, but it offers no added protection from UV light.

Ephelis (freckle)

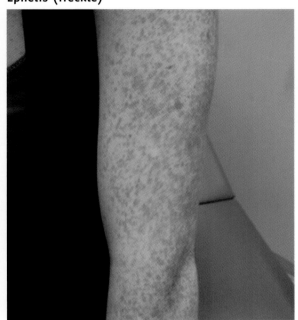

An *ephelis* is commonly known as a *freckle* and first appears during childhood in fair-skinned individuals, presumably developing after sun exposure. When sun exposure is discontinued, the ephelides will typically fade or may even disappear. They represent an increase in melanin production in response to UV radiation exposure. It may be difficult to distinguish clinically between an ephelis and solar lentigo.

- Common on the central face and first noted in childhood
- More prominent after exposure to sunlight, fading after cessation of sunlight exposure
- Familial inheritance and more commonly seen in fair-skinned individuals

Notes

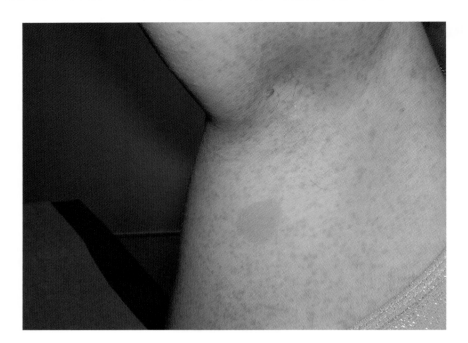

11. A 13-year-old girl presents to your clinic with the chief complaint of several red lumps on her back, arms, legs, and forehead which have been growing in number for 2 months. She adds that she has had coffee-colored marks on her skin since she was a toddler. Her past medical history is significant for a learning disability and recent onset of puberty. On physical exam the patient is Tanner stage 2 in breast and pubic hair development. She has eight café au lait spots on her trunk, numerous neurofibromas over her body, and axillary freckling. She is diagnosed with neurofibromatosis 1 (NF1). Which of the following can be used regarding management of this condition?

A. Imaging of the brain, orbits, chest, spine
B. Eye exam
C. Genetic counseling
D. Surgical removal of dermal neurofibromas
E. Spine exam
F. All of the above

11. **The answer is F: All of the above.** This patient exhibits three of the diagnostic criteria for NF1: 1) Six or more café au lait spots; 2) two or more neurofibromas; 3) freckling in axillary/inguinal region; 4) optic gliomas; 5) two or more iris hamaratomas (Lisch nodules); 6) bony lesions (sphenoid dysplasia/pseudoarthroses); 7) first-degree relative with NF1. Only two of these criteria are needed for diagnosis of NF1. Patients should be referred to NF specialists who can use imaging, usually in the setting of neurologic deficits, to assess for gliomas, sphenoid dysplasia, pseudoarthroses, and spinal lesions. An annual ophthalmological exam is needed to assess for optic pathway gliomas and, to a lesser extent, Lisch nodules. The spine should also be evaluated regularly for signs of scoliosis. Dermal neurofibromas can be surgically removed for cosmetic reasons or for malignant degeneration. Finally all NF patients should receive genetic counseling, as this is an autosomal dominant disorder with 50% chance of inheritance in their offspring (**F**).

Neurofibromatosis

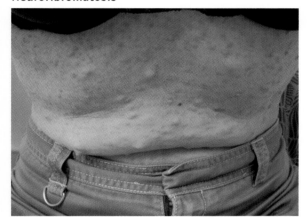

This patient has multiple skin-colored, soft papules and pedunculated nodules on her abdomen. These neurofibromatous lesions are seen in association with neurofibromatosis (NF), an autosomal dominant disease characterized by changes in the skin, nervous system, endocrine glands, and bones. Central nervous system (CNS) involvement occurs in 10% of patients with NF and consists of benign lesions including acoustic neuromas, meningiomas, optic glioma, and in some cases astrocytomas. Thus neurologic signs and symptoms should be approached with a high index of suspicion. Pheochromocytomas occur in 1% of patients, causing severe hypertension. Note café au lait (CAL) macules on abdomen, also a skin finding associated with NF.

- NF1: two or more of the following: six CAL spots (> 15 mm in adults), two neurofibromas, freckling in the axila or inguinal area, optic glioma, two Lisch nodules, osseous abnormality, and a first-degree relative with NF1
- NF2: bilateral acoustic neuromas, a first-degree relative with NF2, and bilateral acoustic neuromas; or any two of the following: neurofibromas, meningiomas, gliomas, or schwannoma
- NF2 features include seizures, skin nodules, and CAL spots.

✎ *Notes* _____

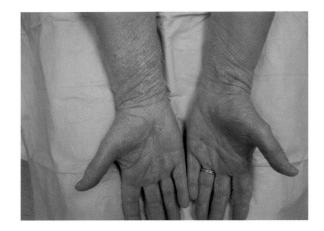

12. A 34-year-old woman presents with thin-walled, fluid-filled blisters over her trunk and extremities. The blisters easily rupture. Her temperature on arrival is 102° F, and her blood pressure is 85/50. You note peeling skin over her palms and soles. The woman was treated 3 weeks ago for a urinary tract infection. The woman takes oral contraceptive pills, but she takes no other medications. Her last menstrual period just ended, and she used a new superabsorbent brand of tampons. What is the cause of this syndrome?

A. Bacterial-released exotoxins
B. Bacterial-released endotoxins
C. Medication reaction
D. Postviral syndrome
E. Antibodies directed against desmoglein molecules

13. A 33-year-old woman presents to the emergency department (ED) with sudden onset fever, chills, vomiting, diarrhea, muscle aches, and a diffuse rash. You are incredibly busy and have not had a chance to see this patient when the nurse alerts you that she has developed severe hypotension and is beginning to decompensate. You start supportive therapy and begin to take a history. She cogently asks you if you think this has anything to do with the sponge that she uses for contraception. She had placed the sponge a week ago and recalls that she forgot to take it out. Which of the following is the most likely cause of her symptoms?

A. Bacterial endotoxins
B. Viral syndrome
C. Allergic reaction
D. Bacterial exotoxins
E. Autoimmune reaction

12. **The answer is A: Bacterial-released exotoxins.** This woman has toxic shock syndrome (TSS), likely due to her use of superabsorbent tampons. TSS is caused by bacterial exotoxins (**A**). Most typically the exotoxins are released by *Staphylococcus aureus*, but can also be due to group A streptococcus. These exotoxins cause detachment within the epidermal layer. Bacterial endotoxins (**B**) are most often associated with gram-negative bacteria, which do not play a role in TSS. Medications (**C**) and a reaction to a viral infection (**D**), such as HSV, are common causes of Stevens-Johnson syndrome (SJS), which classically involveds the mucous membranes and oral mucosa. Antibodies directed against desmoglein molecules (**E**) causes pemphigus vulgaris.

13. **The answer is D: Bacterial exotoxins.** This patient is likely suffering from TSS due to the use of an intravaginal contraceptive device (sponge, an older form of contraception). Menstruating women, women using intravaginal contraceptive devices, people who have undergone nasal surgery, and persons with postoperative staphylococcal wound infections are all at risk for TSS. TSS is caused by bacterial exotoxins (**D**). Fever, chills, vomiting, diarrhea, and rapid, severe hypotension are characteristic of the initial course of TSS. Desquamation, particularly on the palms and soles, can occur 1-2 weeks after onset of the illness. Bacterial endotoxins (**A**) are most often associated with gram-negative bacteria, which do not play a role in TSS. Viral syndromes (**B**) and allergic reactions (**C**) are common causes of SJS, which classically involves the mucous membranes and oral mucosa. TSS is not due to an autoimmune reaction (**E**).

Toxic Shock (Staph Scalded Skin)

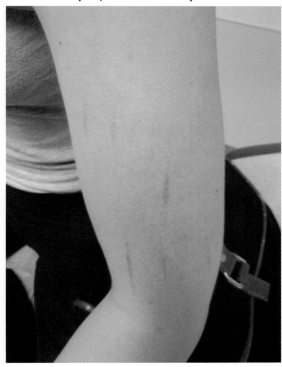

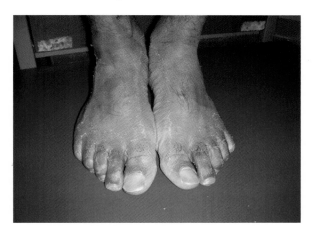

Toxic shock syndrome (TSS) is a rare, life-threatening complication of bacterial infection that has been most often associated with the use of superabsorbent tampons. Often TSS results from toxins produced by *S. aureus*, but it may also be produced by toxins produced by group A streptococcus. *S. aureus* releases epidermolytic exotoxins A and B, which cause detachment within the epidermal layer. These exotoxins are proteases that cleave desmoglein 1, which normally holds the granulosum and spinosum layers together. TSS presents with thin-walled, fluid-filled blisters that easily rupture. Symptoms may also include fever, low blood pressure, vomiting, diarrhea, or a rash, which may lead to desquamation (especially of the palms and soles).

- Caused by exotoxins
- Detachment within epidermal layer
- Treat with antibiotics and supportive care
- Thin-walled blisters and desquamation of skin (particularly hands and soles)

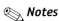
Notes

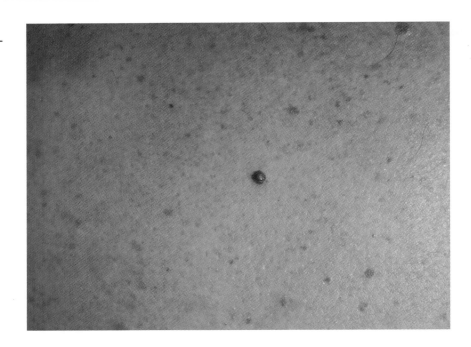

14. A 54-year-old man is in the clinic for an annual visit. During the physical examination, he inquires about multiple red entities present on his chest, upper arms, and back, as shown above. The lesions are cherry red and 1 mm in diameter. They have been there for a few years according to the patient. He has no other health complaints and no significant past medical history. What is the best next step in workup for this patient?

A. Investigation for a visceral adenocarcinoma
B. Biopsies of the lesions to rule out malignancy
C. Mohs procedure for removal
D. Elective laser removal or electrocoagulation
E. Wide local excision

14. **The answer is D: Elective laser removal or electrocoagulation.** This patient has a normal finding of cherry angiomas, which represent benign vascular lesions that are more common with increasing age. The histology of the lesions consists of dilated capillaries and an edematous stroma with homogenization of collagen. They are extremely common in the elderly and have no clinical significance (**A, B**). However, lesions that generate cosmetic concern may be treated with laser therapy or electrocoagulation (**D**). These findings do not warrant more invasive treatment (**C, E**).

Cherry Hemangioma

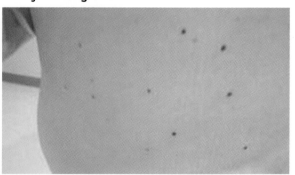

Cherry hemangiomas (or cherry angiomas) are common, asymptomatic, domed vascular lesions that vary in color from bright red to violaceous or black. They are found typically on the trunk, appearing around age 30 and increasing in numbers with age. They have no clinical significance but may pose a cosmetic concern. If desired, they can be treated with laser removal or electrocoagulation.

- Often less than 3 mm in diameter; some smaller lesions are only distinguished from petechiae by their permanence.
- Histology consisting of numerous dilated capillaries lined by flattened endothelium, edematous stroma, and homogenized collagen
- Numbers increase with age but have no clinical significance.

Notes

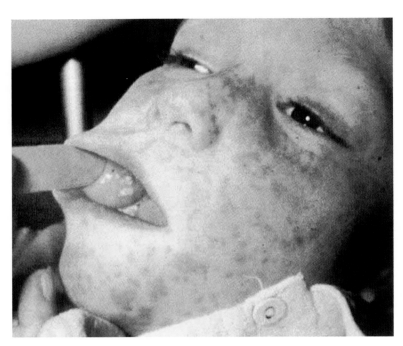

15. A 12-year-old immigrant boy from Brazil presents to the clinic with 5 days of cough, conjunctivitis, fever, and runny nose. His mother brought him in today, alarmed by a rash that began on his head and progressed over his face and neck down his arms to his hands. His medical chart is significant only for absent MMR and Tdap vaccinations. On physical exam a diffuse erythematous, maculopapular rash is noted on his face, neck, chest, and upper extremities. On the buccal mucosa of the inner cheeks, bluish-white spots are noted on erythematous bases bilaterally at the level of the first molars. Which is/are the best treatment option(s) at this time?

A. Antiviral therapy
B. Vitamin A
C. Supportive care
D. Penicillin G
E. All of the above

16. A 3-year-old girl who has no vaccination records presents to an emergency Saturday clinic with a fever, constant cough, runny nose, conjunctivitis, diarrhea, and vomiting for 3 days. On exam the patient is febrile and appears acutely sick with cervical and occipital lymphadenopathy. On oral exam bluish-white spots surrounded by red are noted on the buccal mucosa of the inner cheeks. A clinical diagnosis of measles is made. Supportive care is begun. The next day the patient develops a maculopapular rash on her forehead, which erupts down her face, neck, trunk, and reaches her palms and soles. In discussing the course of the disease you tell her mother that in terms of acute complications, otitis media (AOM) is the most likely, and pneumonia is the most serious. Which of the following is/are known complications of her disease?

A. Subacute sclerosing panencephalitis
B. Diarrhea
C. Death
D. All of the above

15. **The answer is C: Supportive care.** This patient with measles virus has the characteristic exanthem (maculopapular rash starting on the forehead and progressing down the face, neck, trunk, and extremities) after 2-4 days of cough, coryza, and fever. Koplik spots (bluish-white spots on red) develop on the buccal mucosa prior to the onset of the rash and are pathognomonic for measles. Measles IgM antibody is confirmatory. The best treatment in the immunocompetent patient is supportive care: hydration, antipyretics, and maintenance of oxygenation (**C**). Vitamin A is useful if the patient has symptoms of deficiency, malabsorption, malnutrition, or immunosuppression. Ribavirin antiviral could be used with an immunocompromised patient. Antibiotics are not indicated.

16. **The answer is D: All of the above.** This patient has measles due to lack of proper vaccination. Koplik spots (bluish-white spots on red on the buccal mucosa) occurring 1-4 days before the exanthem are pathognomonic for measles. Acutely the leading cause of death is pneumonia. AOM is the most common complication. Diarrhea can lead to dehydration. Subacute sclerosing panencephalitis is a rare, chronic form of measles infection in the CNS, causing fatal neurodegeneration 7-13 years following initial infection (**D**). All of these complications can be avoided with proper MMR vaccination. Side effects of vaccination (fever, injection site rash, and rarely febrile seizure and thrombocytopenia) are minimal considering the risk of complications with measles infection.

Koplik Spots

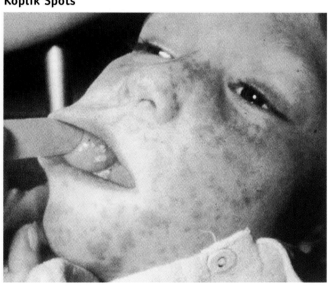

Koplik spots emerge 1 to 2 days before the characteristic erythematous maculopapular rash. They first appear as 1- to 3-mm blue papules with gray-white centers on the buccal mucosa and are pathognomonic for measles infection.

- Pathognomonic for measles infection
- Appear as 1- to 3-mm blue papules with gray-white centers on the buccal mucosa
- Precede the appearance of the maculopapular rash by 1 to 2 days

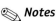 *Notes*

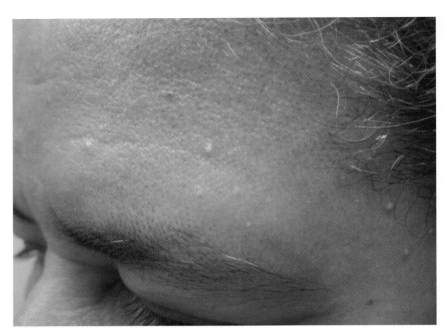

17. A 43-year-old man presents with complaints of lesions around his eyes. He notes that the lesions have been present for a couple of years and have not changed in size, shape, or color. You note that the lesions are 1 mm, raised and non-fluid–filled. What primary skin lesion does this patient have?

A. Macule
B. Papule
C. Patch
D. Plaque
E. Nodule

18. A 10-year-old girl with no significant past medical history is brought to her pediatrician due to several itchy lesions on her abdomen and buttocks. She notes that they have been present for the past couple of months and seem to appear and resolve in different spots. She denies any recent travel or sick contacts but does note that she has a cat who sleeps with her at night. On physical exam, the lesions are 4 mm, raised, erythematous and non-fluid–filled. How would you characterize this patient's primary skin lesion?

A. Macule
B. Patch
C. Plaque
D. Nodule
E. Papule

17. **The answer is B: Papule.** This patient has a papule (**B**) because it is raised, solid, and less than 5 mm. Macules (**A**) are flat lesions less than 10 mm in diameter. A patch (**C**) is a larger nonpalpable lesion greater than 10 mm. Plaques (**D**) are elevated plateau-like palpable lesions greater than 1 cm. Nodules (**E**) are morphologically similar to papules, but they are greater than 1 cm in both width and depth. They are most frequently centered in the dermis or subcutaneous fat.

18. **The answer is E: Papule.** This patient presents with several pruritic, erythematous papules (**E**) likely secondary to flea bites from her cat. A papule is a solid, elevated lesion less than 5 mm in which a significant portion projects above the plane of the surrounding skin. A macule (**A**) is any flat lesion of less than 10 mm in diameter that is even with the surface of surrounding skin and differs in color from the surrounding skin or mucous membrane. Patches (**B**) are larger, flat nonpalpable lesions measuring greater than 10 mm in size. Plaques (**C**) are elevated palpable lesions greater than 10 mm. A nodule (**D**) is a solid, round, or ellipsoidal palpable lesion with a diameter larger than 5 mm. Nodules are differentiated from papules and plaques by depth of involvement and/or substantive palpability.

Papule

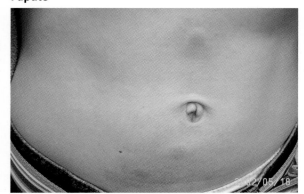

A *papule* is a primary skin lesion defined by a palpable, solid, well-circumscribed elevation of skin measuring less than 5 mm in diameter.

- Palpable lesion less than 5 mm
- Primary skin lesion
- May be associated with secondary features such as crusts or scales

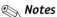

✎ *Notes*

_____

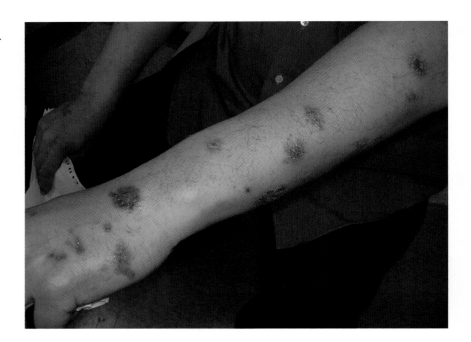

19. A 50-year-old man with a history of atopic dermatitis presents to the clinic with golden-crusted, erythematous, weeping lesions on his left arm. He is afebrile and otherwise healthy. Gram stain of the fluid reveals gram-positive cocci in chains, and culture of the weeping area grows group A streptococci after 24 hours. What is the next appropriate step in the clinical management of this patient?

A. IV penicillin and vancomycin
B. Warm compresses and IV penicillin
C. Second generation cephalosporin
D. Topical mupirocin ointment after removal of dirt, crusts, and debris with soap and water
E. Prophylactic ampicillin for all close contacts

20. A 17-year-old woman presents to the clinic with 3 days of a perioral, crusty, yellow rash. She says that crusting started at a crack at the corner of her mouth and gradually grew to her chin. On exam a honey-crusted rash is noted at the chin and corners of the mouth with some small unruptured vesicles on erythematous bases. A clinical diagnosis of impetigo is made. Which of the following is/are true regarding this condition?

A. Highly contagious, capable of self-inoculation
B. Can start at site of skin injury or on intact skin
C. Represents an infection with *S. aureus* and/or group A streptococcus
D. Treatment is topical mupirocin ointment
E. All of the above

19. The answer is D: Topical mupirocin ointment after removal of dirt, crusts, and debris with soap and water. This patient has impetigo caused by group A streptococci based on clinical findings and confirmed with Gram stain and culture. Impetigo is a superficial skin infection that very rarely has systemic effects and can be effectively treated with either topical mupirocin ointment or oral penicillin (**D**). Removal of crusts and debris with soap and water is a helpful adjunct. Impetigo is a very contagious, autoinoculable infection. Clinical differentiation between streptococcal and staphylococcal lesions is difficult, and older erosions may contain both types of bacteria. IV antibiotics and prophylaxis of close contacts are not warranted.

20. The answer is E: All of the above. This patient has nonbullous impetigo, which is diagnosed clinically as small vesicles on a red base. As vesicles rupture, an adherent yellow-brown, honey-colored crust forms. Locally additional sites of clustered vesicles will appear as this dermal staphylococcal and/or group A streptococcal infection grows. Areas of skin around the mouth and nose are usual sites. Although not necessary, skin injury as well as preexisting lesions such as eczema or a cold sore can lead to impetigo with the introduction of infectious bacteria. Impetigo is highly contagious and most prominent in younger children. Treatment of this local superficial infection involves isolation and avoidance of physical contact and topical mupirocin ointment (**E**). Systemic antibiotics should be used only for extensive cases of impetigo.

Impetigo

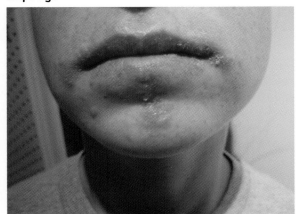

Impetigo is caused by skin infection with either streptococci or staphylococci and appears as crusted superficial erosions that contain purulent material and rupture easily. The lesions may appear as macules, vesicles, bullae, pustules, and honey-colored gummy crusts. Impetigo is a highly contagious infection and individuals can often autoinoculate themselves. The face and other exposed areas are most commonly affected. Gram stain and culture confirm the diagnosis.

- Streptococcal and staphylococcal causes of impetigo are clinically indistinguishable, except for bullous impetigo.
- Preexisting lesions like scabies, zoster, or eczema can predispose patients to the infection.
- Gram stain and culture confirm the diagnosis.

✎ *Notes* _____

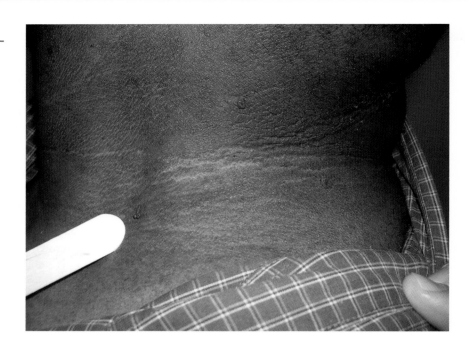

21. A 42-year-old African American man presents to the office for a routine checkup. On examination, he has darkened skin on the back of his neck (shown above), axilla, and elbows, which he states has been there for a few months. He is mildly overweight, but otherwise he has no significant past medical history and presents with no other medical complaints. What is the best next step in this patient's ongoing therapy?

A. Skin biopsy
B. Fasting glucose level
C. CA 125, CEA, and CA 19-9 tumor markers for underlying neoplasm
D. CAT scan of the abdomen and pelvis
E. Reassurance with no further workup

22. A 65-year-old African American man states that multiple areas of his skin have suddenly become darker. He also complains of intermittent epigastric pain and an inability to finish his meals over the last few weeks. He says he "feels full" with minimal food intake and notes that his clothes seem looser. His fasting glucose and hemoglobin A1c are normal. What is the next best step?

A. Topical retinoid
B. Upper endoscopy
C. Skin biopsy
D. Recommend diet and exercise
E. Reassurance with no further workup

21. **The answer is B: Fasting glucose level.** This patient's findings represent the classic presentation for acanthosis nigricans, which consists of hyperkeratosis and hyperpigmentation of the neck, axilla, groin, and other skin folds, especially on flexural surfaces. This condition is most commonly associated with type 2 diabetes mellitus and insulin resistance. Therefore the best initial course of action to take with this patient is to obtain a fasting glucose level (**B**). Although acanthosis nigricans has also been seen in patients with adenocarcinomas of the gastrointestinal (GI) and genitourinary tract (**C, D**), especially gastric carcinomas, this is not the most likely etiology of the condition. Typically cases associated with carcinomas have a rapid onset, and the patient in this case has an insidious onset of the disorder. A skin biopsy (**A**) will show typical dermatopathology findings of hyperkeratosis, epidermal papillomatosis, slight acanthosis, and possible increased melanin pigmentation, but it will not provide diagnostic value in revealing the underlying disorder. Choice **E** is incorrect because a diabetes workup is indicated in patients who present with this clinical finding.

22. **The answer is B: Upper endoscopy.** Acanthosis nigricans with rapid onset raises suspicion for malignancy, most commonly gastric carcinoma. Although malignancy is a rare cause of acanthosis nigricans, rapid onset of skin changes, coupled with the patient's symptoms of abdominal pain, early satiety, and weight loss, warrant investigation for gastric cancer with upper endoscopy (**B**). Acanthosis nigricans lesions secondary to insulin resistance (the most common cause) and malignancy are indistinguishable, so skin biopsy (**C**) will not help to identify the underlying cause. A topical medication to improve the cosmetic appearance of the acanthosis nigricans (**A**) and initiation of a diet and exercise program (**D**) may be appropriate if serious causes of acanthosis nigricans are ruled out; however, the patient's symptoms plus the rapid onset of the acanthosis nigricans makes these choices, as well as reassurance (**E**), inappropriate at this time.

Acanthosis Nigricans

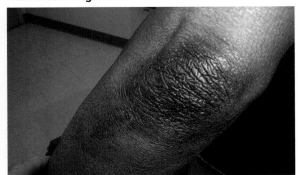

Acanthosis nigricans is a cutaneous marker commonly associated with insulin resistance and less frequently with genetic disorders or malignancy. It is characterized by symmetric, hyperpigmented plaques that typically appear on skin folds, especially the flexural areas.

- Acanthosis nigricans most often has an insidious onset and signifies insulin resistance from any cause, commonly type 2 diabetes mellitus.
- Diagnostic workup initially includes testing for diabetes mellitus and metabolic syndrome. Imaging tests and endoscopy should be used if there is acute onset to rule out malignancy.
- Treatment is targeted to the underlying cause, if identified. Topical keratolytic or topical retinoids may improve acanthosis nigricans, as can weight loss in obese patients.

✎ *Notes*

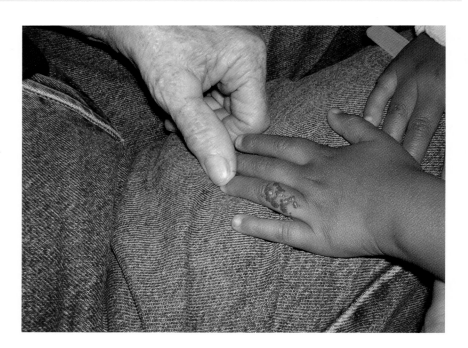

23. A 4-year-old girl presents with a red-purple, raised vascular plaque over her left fourth digit. The lesion appeared a couple weeks after she was born. It grew rapidly for a period of time, but has been stable for about a year. What is the next step in treatment?

A. Surgical excision and biopsy
B. Laser surgery
C. Cryosurgery
D. Systemic glucocorticoids
E. No treatment

24. A first-time mother brings her 1-month-old infant to her pediatrician concerned by a growing plaque on her left buttock. Her mom comments that there was a red mark present at birth but is concerned that this mark has not resolved and has in fact continued to grow and now demonstrates a raised, vascular appearance. Which of the following is the best advice for this concerned mother?

A. Advise the mother to take her infant to a dermatologist to remove this lesion before 24 months of age.
B. Reassurance that most of these lesions resolve spontaneously
C. Biopsy of the lesion to rule out a malignant vascular neoplasm
D. Reassurance that while this lesion will likely be permanent it is not malignant in nature
E. Advise the use of topical corticosteroids to speed resolution.

23. **The answer is E: No treatment.** This lesion is a strawberry hemangioma (also called an *infantile hemangioma* or a *capillary hemangioma*). The best treatment for these lesions is to let them resolve spontaneously (**E**). About 60% resolve by age 5, and 90% are gone by age 9. Treatment is only necessary if the lesion blocks vision, is in the way of the nostrils, or if ulceration occurs. If surgery is necessary, laser surgery (**B**) or cryosurgery (**C**) may be indicated. Surgical excision and biopsy (**A**) is not indicated in this case as the diagnosis can be made clinically. Systemic glucocorticoids (**D**) may be initiated if treatment is indicated, but spontaneous resolution generally gives the best results.

24. **The answer is B: Reassurance that most of these lesions resolve spontaneously.** This lesion is most likely a strawberry hemangioma and will resolve spontaneously (**B**). Biopsy (**C**) or treatment (**D**) is not necessary, and clinical diagnosis is usually sufficient. Topical corticosteroids have not been demonstrated to be beneficial (**E**), and referral to a dermatologist is not indicated at this time.

Strawberry Hemangioma

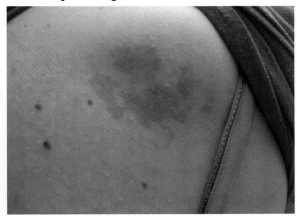

Strawberry hemangiomas (also called *capillary hemangiomas* or *infantile hemangiomas*) are superficial vascular tumors which appear as raised, red, lumpy areas of flesh anywhere on the body, although the majority occur on the head or neck. These hemangiomas are clonal proliferations of endothelial cells. They usually appear about 1-4 weeks after birth and may grow rapidly before stopping and then slowly fading. About 60% resolve by age 5, and about 90% are gone by age 9. Women are more often affected than males. The incidence is increased in preterm infants. No treatment is necessary unless the lesion blocks vision or is in the way of the nostrils.

- Rapid growth phase followed by spontaneous involution
- Increased incidence in women and in preterm infants
- Resolve spontaneously
- Intervention necessary if ulceration occurs or if the lesion causes functional impairment

✎ *Notes*

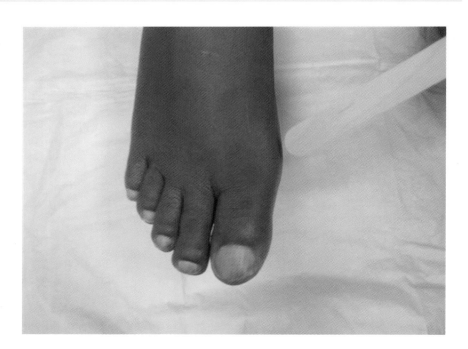

25. A 40-year-old man comes to the clinic complaining of pain at the base of his right great toe, which has been going on since he woke up. He has pain while ambulating and had trouble putting on his shoes. He has hypertension controlled on hydrochlorothiazide (HCTZ) and lisinopril and takes atorvastatin for hyperlipidemia. He drinks 1-2 beers each night after dinner. On examination he has a BMI of 30 and stable vital signs. He has swelling and erythema at the base of the right hallux, and he pulls his foot away briskly in pain when this area is palpated. Needle aspiration of the area is performed, and blood work is drawn for serum uric acid. What change(s) may be helpful in this patient to prevent future gouty attacks?

A. Weight loss
B. Cessation of alcohol consumption
C. Discontinuation of the diuretic
D. Staying well hydrated
E. All of the above

26. A 70-year-old African American woman presents to clinic with a painful bump on her finger. Her past medical history is significant for alcohol abuse. On exam there is an inflamed Heberden node on her right first distal interphalangeal (DIP) joint that is extremely tender to palpation. Labs reveal elevated erythrocyte sedimentation rate (ESR) and elevated uric acid levels. Aspirate from the nodule demonstrates negatively birefringent needle-shaped crystals and a white blood count (WBC) of $12,000 \times 10^3/\mu L$. A diagnosis of acute gouty attack is made. What is/are an appropriate treatment(s) of gout?

A. Colchicine
B. Cessation of alcohol consumption
C. Nonsteroidal antiinflammatory drug (NSAID)
D. Corticosteroid injection
E. All of the above

25. **The answer is E: All of the above.** This patient is suffering from acute gouty arthritis. The most commonly affected location is the first metatarsophalangeal joint, and treatment of an acute attack is aimed at analgesia and antiinflammatory measures. Needle aspiration of synovial fluid from the affected joint will help to rule out other causes (e.g., septic arthritis) and show the characteristic monosodium urate crystals on compensated polarized light microscopy. The crystals are needle-shaped and appear yellow when parallel to the axis of rotation of the compensator and blue when perpendicular. While allopurinol therapy in the intercritical period between attacks may lessen morbidity from gout, issues like obesity, hyperlipidemia, diabetes, alcoholism, smoking, and hydration take priority. Lifestyle changes can have a positive effect on a patient's prognosis after the first attack (**E**), because all these factors affect purine and/or uric acid metabolism in the body.

26. **The answer is E: All of the above.** This patient is suffering from an acute tophaceous gouty arthritis. First-line treatment includes NSAIDs (indomethacin, naproxen). Intraarticular steroid injections can offer more immediate relief and have no systemic side effects. Colchicine can decrease inflammation if used early in a gouty attack. Both allopurinol and cessation of alcohol are effective as long-term therapies in patients with hyperuricemia and recurrent gouty attacks (**E**).

Gout

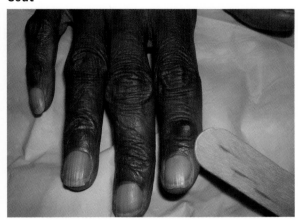

Gout is characterized by a group of heterogeneous conditions that result in the deposition of monosodium urate crystals in the synovial fluid, usually with associated hyperuricemia. It is typically characterized by four stages: asymptomatic hyperuricemia, acute gouty arthritis, intercritical gout (between attacks), and chronic tophaceous gout. Leukocytosis and elevated ESR are often present during acute attacks. Treatment revolves around analgesia and reduction in inflammation in the acute setting with NSAIDs, colchicine, and corticosteroids. Chronic treatment includes xanthine oxidase inhibitors like allopurinol.

- Acute gouty arthritis typically presents in the middle years and affects a single joint in the lower extremities, most commonly the first metatarsophalangeal joint.
- Affected joints are erythematous and extremely tender to palpation.
- Chronic tophaceous gout rarely grants patients periods without symptoms. Urate crystals can be found in the soft tissues, cartilage, and tendons.

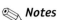

✎ *Notes*

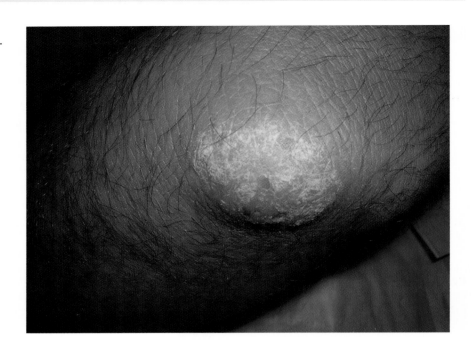

27. A 45-year-old man presents with symmetric lesions over his knees. The lesions appear as a silvery scale on an erythematous base. The man reports that he is otherwise healthy. You note that slight scratching of the scaly lesions results in punctate bleeding points. What is the most likely cause of these lesions?

A. Trauma
B. Lichen simplex chronicus
C. Seborrheic dermatitis
D. Atopic dermatitis
E. Psoriasis

28. A 38-year-old man presents complaining of a rash on his leg and chronic pain in his fingers and lower back for the past 6 months. He has no significant medical history but does note that his father suffered from something similar. On physical exam you note lesions with a silvery scale on an erythematous base throughout the patient's left leg and with passive motion of the DIP joints of his right hand as well as mild tenderness to palpation at the sacroiliac joint. You also identify that the patient has pitting on the nails of his fingers. What would be the next best step in diagnosing this patient's disease?

A. Skin biopsy of lesions on leg
B. MRI of lumbar spine
C. No further tests, the diagnosis can be made solely on clinical findings
D. Check for human leukocyte antigen B27 (HLA-B27)
E. Check uric acid level in urine

27. The answer is E: Psoriasis. Psoriatic lesions typically occur on extensor surfaces and often exhibit Koebner phenomenon and Auspitz sign (slight scratching of the scaly lesions results in punctate bleeding points). Although bony prominences may be damaged during trauma (**A**), a description of a silver scale on an erythematous base is a classic description of psoriasis. Lichen simplex chronicus (**B**) occurs due to habitually scratching an area of skin. The skin eventually thickens and darkens. These changes are called *lichenification*. Seborrheic dermatitis (**C**) causes red or golden scaly patches of skin around areas with oily skin, such as the ears, eyebrows, scalp, and nasolabial fold. Atopic dermatitis (**D**) typically affects flexor surfaces and can lead to lichenification.

28. The answer is C: No further tests, the diagnosis can be made solely on clinical findings. This patient has the signs and symptoms of psoriatic arthritis, an inflammatory arthritis that characteristically occurs in individuals with psoriasis. A diagnosis can be made based on clinical findings (**C**) of psoriasis and arthropathy along with nail changes ranging from pitting, horizontal ridging, onycholysis, yellowish discoloration, or dystrophic hyperkeratosis. A skin biopsy (**A**) may be helpful if one is unsure of the psoriasis on this patient's leg. However, it would not help to characterize his arthropathy. An MRI of the lumbar spine (**B**) may show nonspecific changes that would not be useful for a diagnosis. Although HLA-B27 (**D**) is found in 50%-70% of patients with axial disease, it would not be useful to rule out psoriatic arthritis in this case. Uric acid (**E**) levels may be elevated in the presence of extensive psoriasis. However, this is a nonspecific finding and would not help diagnosis this patient's disease.

Psoriasis

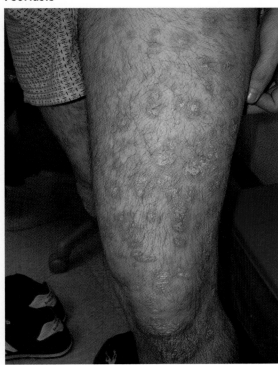

Psoriasis is a common chronic skin disorder typically characterized by inflamed, edematous skin lesions covered with a silvery white scale. Plaque psoriasis is the most common type and is characterized by symmetric patches on the scalp, trunk, and limbs. The most common sites are the extensor surfaces of the limbs. Guttate psoriasis is characterized by small red dots and frequently appears after an upper respiratory infection. Nail psoriasis may cause pits in the nails, which may become yellow and thickened, eventually separating from the nail bed. Psoriatic arthritis affects approximately 10% of those with skin symptoms. The arthritis is usually in the hands, feet, and larger joints. It produces stiffness, pain, and progressive joint damage. Psoriatic lesions may demonstrate Auspitz sign (slight scratching of the scaly lesions revealing punctate bleeding points) or Koebner phenomenon (lesions occurring in areas of irritation/ scratching, such as the pant line). The diagnosis is usually clinical. If there is a questionable diagnosis, a punch biopsy may be performed. Treatment options include PUVA, topical retinoids, and cytotoxic agents such as methotrexate and cyclosporine.

- Extensor surfaces
- Silver scales on an erythematous base
- Symmetric
- Auspitz sign
- Koebner phenomenon
- Abnormal T lymphocyte function

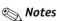

Notes

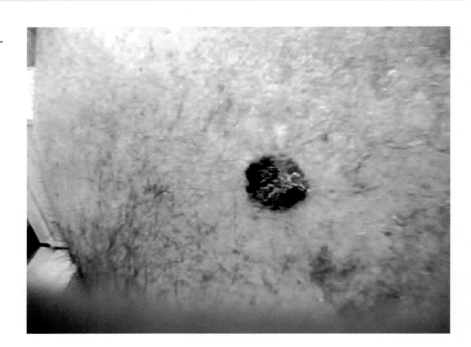

29. A 65-year-old man presents with a thick dome-shaped lesion on his scalp. The lesion is blue-black, 7 mm in size, and he noted that the lesion sometimes bleeds when he irritates the area. What is the most likely diagnosis?

A. Benign nevi
B. Basal cell carcinoma
C. Squamous cell carcinoma
D. Melanoma
E. Actinic keratosis

30. A 40-year-old man presents with a black, raised lesion on his upper back. The patient noticed that the lesion has almost doubled in size over the past 6 months. On physical exam the lesion is 1 cm, nontender, and asymmetric with irregular borders. What is the correct way to characterize this lesion?

A. Nodular melanoma
B. Superficial spreading melanoma
C. Lentigo maligna
D. Acral lentiginous melanoma
E. Actinic keratosis

29. **The answer is D: Melanoma.** This patient has findings of melanoma (**D**) as indicated by the size, color, border, and asymmetry. The lesion's characteristics are concerning for a malignant process rather than a benign nevi (**A**). Basal cell carcinoma (**B**) is the most common skin cancer. They are often slowly growing, raised papular lesions that rarely metastasize. Basal cell carcinomas may be translucent or pearly with rolled borders or telangiectasia. Squamous cell carcinoma (**C**) is the second most common skin cancer and usually occurs in sun-exposed areas. It is characterized by red, scaly skin that may ulcerate. Actinic keratosis (**E**) is a rough, scaly, dark brown or pink patch that appears after years of sun exposure. A small number of actinic keratoses eventually develop into squamous cell carcinomas.

30. **The answer is A: Nodular melanoma.** This lesion is a nodular melanoma (**A**), the second most common melanoma subtype, accounting for 15%-30% of all melanomas. Nodular melanomas are remarkable for rapid evolution, often arising over several weeks to months, and typically appear as uniformly dark black-blue lesions with irregular borders and measuring over 6 mm in size. Superficial spreading melanomas (**B**) are the most common subtype and account for around 70% of all cutaneous melanomas. Classically, these subtypes appear with asymmetry, irregular scalloped borders, and often various shades of color. They do not project prominently from the skin and are often nonpalpable. Lentigo maligna (**C**) displays asymmetry, poorly defined irregular borders, and is generally a flat, slowly enlarging, brown, freckle-like macule. Acral lentiginous melanoma (**D**) only constitutes 2%-8% of all melanomas in Caucasians but up to 60%-72% in African Americans. The most common sites are the sole, palm, and subungual locations, and lesions can appear brown, black, tan, or red. Actinic keratosis (**E**) occurs in fair-skinned older individuals with extensive sun exposure. These lesions are typically 2-6 mm in size and appear as erythematous, flat, rough, or scaly papules.

Melanoma

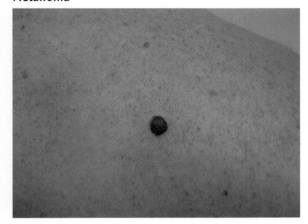

Melanoma is a malignant tumor of melanocytes found predominantly in the skin. It is less common than many other types of skin cancer, but accounts for 75% of skin cancer–related deaths. There are four main types of melanomas. Superficial spreading melanomas are the most common and are usually flat and irregular in shape and color. Nodular melanomas usually start as a raised area. Lentigo maligna melanomas usually occur in the elderly on sun-damaged areas such as the face, neck, and arms. Acral lentiginous melanomas usually occur on the palms, soles, or under the nails and are more common in African Americans.

- Treatment includes surgical removal of the tumor, adjuvant treatment, chemotherapy and immunotherapy, or radiation therapy.
- Dermatopathology: hyperplasia and proliferation of melanocytes in a single-file pattern in the basal cell layer
- ABCDE
  - **A**symmetrical skin lesion
  - **B**order of lesion is irregular
  - **C**olor: melanomas usually have multiple colors
  - **D**iameter: moles greater than 6 mm are more likely to be melanomas
  - **E**nlarging: enlarging or evolving

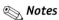 *Notes*

_____

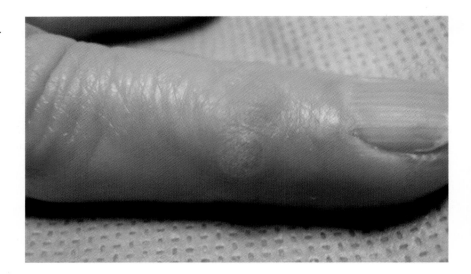

31. A 43-year-old man presents with a well-demarcated, rough, slightly raised lesion on his finger. The lesion has been present for about 3 months. What is the cause of this lesion?

A. Virus
B. Fungus
C. Bacteria
D. Cellular overgrowth
E. Cellular necrosis

32. A 24-year-old man comes to your office complaining of an uncomfortable bump on his index finger (shown above). This lesion has been present for the past 2 years despite many attempts at home removal. The lesion is rough, slightly raised, and has a cauliflower-like appearance upon closer inspection. Which of the following is the most appropriate treatment for this patient's condition?

A. Cryotherapy
B. Surgical excision
C. Soak lesion in hot water for 10-30 minutes
D. Carbon dioxide laser therapy
E. Photodynamic therapy

31. **The answer is A: Virus.** This man has a lesion consistent with a verrucae, or wart. Warts are caused by the human papillomavirus (HPV) (**A**). They are classified based on their shape and the area of the body affected. There are several strains of HPV. Verrucae are not a fungal (**B**) or bacterial (**C**) infection. They are not caused by cellular overgrowth (**D**) or necrosis (**E**). Common warts often disappear on their own in a few months but may last years and may also recur. Treatment options include cryotherapy or salicylic acid.

32. **The answer is A: Cryotherapy.** The lesion on this patient's finger is most likely a verrucae or wart due to a viral infection with human papillomavirus. The most appropriate treatment listed is cryotherapy (**A**). Surgical excision is rarely necessary (**B**). Soaking the lesion in hot water for 10-30 minutes daily for 6 weeks may aid in resolution, but a one-time soak (**C**) is unlikely to be beneficial. Carbon dioxide laser therapy (**D**) and photodynamic therapy (**E**) should be reserved for lesions that fail initial cryotherapy or salicylic acid treatment.

Verrucae

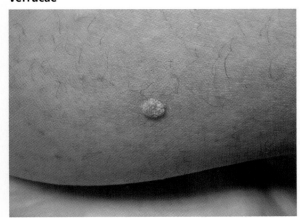

Verrucae, also called warts, are well-demarcated, rough, hard nodules or plaques with an irregular surface caused by the HPV. They typically disappear after a few months but can last years and can recur. Warts are classified based on their shape and the area of the body affected. Common warts are raised and rough and are most common on the hands. Other types of warts include flat warts, filiform warts, plantar warts, genital warts, or periungual warts. Cryotherapy or salicylic acid can also be used to remove the lesion.

- Caused by HPV
- Treated with cryotherapy or salicylic acid

✎ *Notes*
_____

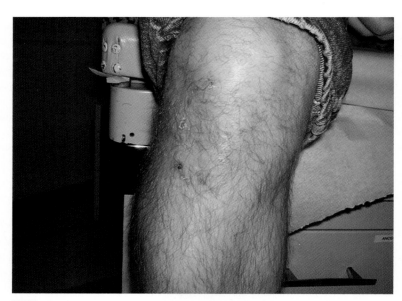

33. A 27-year-old man presents to the clinic complaining of a severely pruritic rash that recently erupted on his skin. He has never experienced a similar rash and appears anxious for symptomatic relief. He denies any GI complaints and has no significant past medical history. Physical examination reveals erythematous patches and plaques with crusts and erosions in a symmetric pattern on his elbows, knees, dorsa of the hands, upper back, and gluteal crease. A biopsy of one of the lesions shows subepidermal vesicles at the tips of dermal papillae with intravesicular neutrophil collections. Immunofluorescent staining of a biopsy from normal-appearing skin reveals granular IgA deposits. Which of the following statements regarding this patient's diagnosis is/are true?

A. The rash will respond rapidly to dapsone.
B. This patient is at increased risk for developing GI lymphoma.
C. Strict adherence to a gluten-free diet helps to decrease exacerbations and resolve the rash.
D. All of the above

34. A 32-year-old woman presents to your office with a 1-year history of a pruritic rash on her back and extensor surfaces of both arms and legs. Her past medical history is significant for iron-deficiency anemia and chronic steatorrhea causing a 30-pound weight loss over the past year. Physical exam is significant for pale conjunctivae and small groups of vesicles with crusting on erythematous plaques present symmetrically on her back, buttocks, and extensor surfaces. A biopsy from healthy skin around the lesions shows IgA deposits at the dermal-epidermal junction, confirming a diagnosis of dermatitis herpetiformis (DH). Blood tests are positive for antiendomysial and antitissue transglutaminase antibodies, and biopsy of the small bowel shows atrophic villi and intraepithelial lymphocytosis, confirming associated celiac disease. In the treatment of this patient, which of the following has been shown to decrease the symptoms of both autoimmune disorders long term?

A. Dapsone
B. Prednisone
C. Gluten-free diet
D. Sulphapyridine
E. Tetracycline

33. **The answer is D: All of the above.** This patient is experiencing DH, which presents as an intensely pruritic, chronic papulovesicular eruption symmetrically on the extensor surfaces. While these patients have a gluten-sensitive enteropathy, fewer than 10% are symptomatic. This enteropathy, however, places them at higher risk for developing GI lymphoma. The rash responds rapidly to sulfa drugs, especially dapsone, and to a gluten-free diet, which must be maintained to prevent cutaneous disease. Thus all answer options are true (**D**). A biopsy from normal appearing skin that shows granular IgA deposits is diagnostic. Dapsone use may be limited by dose-related hemolytic anemia and idiopathic neuropathy.

34. **The answer is C: Gluten-free diet.** This patient exhibits symptoms of malabsorption (iron-deficiency anemia, steatorrhea, and weight loss). Because DH is unique to gluten-sensitive enteropathy, celiac disease is the most likely and proven cause of this malabsorption. In treating this patient, she should be tested and treated for deficiencies of fat-soluble vitamins (A, D, E, K), calcium, folate, iron, and vitamin B_{12}. She should also be evaluated for osteoporosis. Dapsone and other sulfa drugs (sulphapyridine) are used for immediate relief and control of DH. Additional therapies for DH include tetracycline and prednisone. However, initiation and maintenance of a gluten-free diet is the long-term therapy for both DH and celiac disease (**C**). In celiac disease, symptom relief may take days to weeks, and histologic recovery may take months to years on a gluten-free diet. After 6 months of strict gluten- and gliadin-free diet, sulfa drugs may be dose-decreased or discontinued in treatment of DH.

Dermatitis Herpetiformis

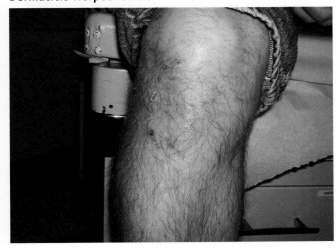

Dermatitis herpetiformis (DH) is a chronic, severely pruritic, papulovesicular eruption that usually follows a symmetric distribution over the extensor surfaces. Histologically, it consists of dermal papillary collections of neutrophils, termed *microabscesses*. Almost all patients with DH have an associated gluten-sensitive enteropathy. It may present at any age and persists indefinitely, with varying severity if the underlying gluten sensitivity is not treated.

- Chronic, recurrent, intensely itchy eruption symmetrically on extensor surfaces of the extremities and trunk; lesions may be vesicles (most common), erythematous papules, urticaria-like plaques, or bullae (infrequently)
- Histologically characterized by papillary neutrophil collections
- Granular IgA deposits in paralesional or normal-appearing skin are diagnostic.
- Rash responds rapidly to dapsone and adherence to a gluten-free diet.

✎ *Notes* _____

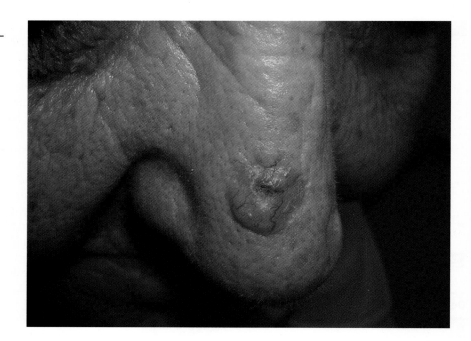

35. An 82-year-old man is brought from a nursing home to your office by his daughter, who is visiting from out of town and became concerned about bleeding from a lump on her father's nose. The patient's memory is poor, and he cannot give a complete history, saying only, "I guess I just never noticed it." He has no complaints, and his past medical history is significant only for Alzheimer's dementia. Physical examination reveals a pearly papule on the nose that has a waxy appearance, central crater with scab, and visible telangiectasia. Multiple actinic keratoses are seen on the face and hands. What is the next appropriate step in this patient's management?

A. Shave or punch biopsy
B. Referral for immediate irradiation
C. Whole body PET scan for staging purposes
D. Three cycles of curettage and electrodesiccation
E. Topical chemotherapy to shrink the lesion before surgical removal

36. A 75-year-old retired fisherman comes in for a routine physical. He points out a spot on his chest that has been present for more than a year. He says it occasionally bleeds and is about the same size as when he first noticed it. The lesion has an ulcerated base covered with a crust. Biopsy reveals atypical basal cells with palisading nuclei. Which of the following is the most likely diagnosis?

A. Squamous cell carcinoma
B. Melanoma
C. Basal cell carcinoma
D. Seborrheic keratosis
E. Actinic keratosis

35. **The answer is A: Shave or punch biopsy.** This patient has basal cell carcinoma. The nodular type, has a characteristic translucent, waxy, or pearly appearance. A shave or punch biopsy is required to confirm the diagnosis (**A**). The lesion can then be treated with excision, curettage, electrodesiccation, or Mohs micrographic surgery. Curettage and electrodesiccation may be curative but leave a broad scar; therefore, these methods should not be used for basal cell carcinoma on the head and neck (**D**). Mohs micrographic surgery is tissue sparing and has the highest cure rate among treatment options. Irradiation may be considered for older patients (> 65 years), but recurrent lesions are aggressive and difficult to treat. Because up to half of patients will develop a second lesion, they should be monitored closely for new or recurrent lesions. Basal cell carcinoma rarely metastatasizes so treatment is local excision. Therefore PET scan for staging purposes, irradiation, and/or chemotherapy, are not part of the workup and treatment (**B, C, E**).

36. **The answer is C: Basal cell carcinoma.** The patient has an ulcerating basal cell carcinoma (**C**). It is common with this type of basal cell carcinoma for the ulcer to be covered with a crust. As with the nodular type, ulcerating basal cell carcinoma lesions are typically translucent and pearly, with peripheral telangiectasia. Basal cell carcinoma is slow growing, with virtually no metastatic potential. Atypical basal cells with palisading nuclei are found on biopsy. Squamous cell carcinoma (**A**) can also ulcerate and crust, but biopsy shows atypical keratinocytes and malignant epidermal cells penetrating the basement membrane. Melanoma (**B**) can also ulcerate, but the lesion in this case is slow growing and shows characteristics of basal cell carcinoma on biopsy. Seborrheic keratosis (**D**) presents as waxy brown papules and plaques, which have a "stuck-on" appearance. Actinic keratoses (**E**) are light, scaly, erythematous lesions. They are a precursor to squamous cell carcinoma.

Basal Cell Carcinoma

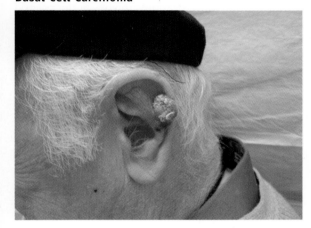

Basal cell carcinoma is the most common skin cancer. It has a characteristic translucent, waxy, or pearly appearance. As the lesion enlarges, it often develops an umbilicated or ulcerated center and peripheral telangiectasia.

- Major risk factor: chronic sunlight exposure
- Tumor is slow growing and locally invasive, aggressive, and destructive
- Metastasis is extremely rare.
- Diagnose clinically; confirm with biopsy
- Treat with excision, curettage, electrodesiccation, or Mohs micrographic surgery

Notes

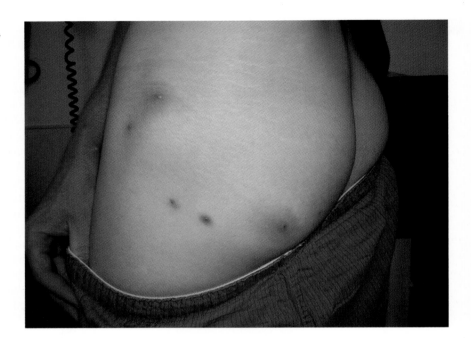

37. A 17-year-old man presents with lesions over his thighs, buttocks, and arms. The lesions appear to have a small raised central white area with an erythematous base and contain necrotic inflammatory cells. How would you describe this patient's lesions?

A. Pustule
B. Vesicle
C. Bullae
D. Nodule
E. Cyst

38. A 4-year-old girl presents to her primary care physician with several itchy lesions over her torso, face, and buttocks. These lesions began 2 days ago. Her mother notes that she is enrolled in daycare where several other children also experienced similar lesions. On physical exam the lesions are 3-5 mm in size and appear as circumscribed, raised lesions with a central whitish, pus-filled area. How would you classify this patient's lesion type?

A. Papule
B. Pustule
C. Nodule
D. Macule
E. Bullae

37. **The answer is A: Pustule.** This patient has pustules (**A**) due to folliculitis. Pustules are small raised lesions filled with cloudy, purulent material (necrotic inflammatory cells). Vesicles (**B**) are circumscribed fluid-containing epidermal elevations measuring less than 1 cm, commonly referred to as *blisters*. Bullae (**C**) are large vesicles and are greater than 1 cm. Nodules (**D**) are greater than 1 cm and are centered in the dermis or subcutaneous fat. Cysts (**E**) are cavities with a closed sac that contain a liquid, semisolid, or solid material.

38. **The answer is B: Pustule.** This patient has pustules (**B**) likely secondary to a varicella infection. Pustules are small raised lesions filled with cloudy, purulent material (necrotic inflammatory cells). Papules (**A**) are solid, elevated lesions measuring less than 0.5 cm in which a significant portion projects above the plane of the surrounding skin. Nodules (**C**) are greater than 1 cm and are centered in the dermis or subcutaneous fat. Macules (**D**) are flat lesions of less than 10 mm in diameter that are even with the surface of surrounding skin and differ in color from the surrounding skin or mucous membrane. Bullae (**E**) are large vesicles greater than 1 cm.

Pustule

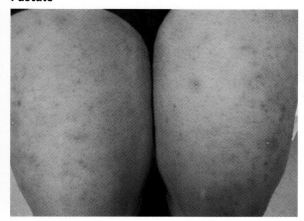

A *pustule* is a small elevation of the skin containing cloudy or purulent material usually consisting of necrotic inflammatory cells or exudate.

- Elevated
- Contains pus (necrotic inflammatory cells)
- May vary in size
- May or may not be related to hair follicles

Notes

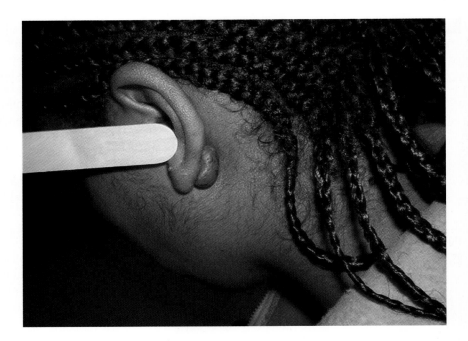

39. A 29-year-old African American woman complains about a growth on the posterior aspect of her earlobe during an office visit. It appeared where she received a second ear piercing during her pregnancy last year and continued to grow even after she removed the earring. She is requesting that it be removed. What are her treatment options?

A. Cryosurgery
B. Excision at the base
C. Topical triamcinolone
D. Wide-margin excision with a skin flap
E. Biopsy to confirm diagnosis

40. A 25-year-old African American patient presents to the clinic with multiple growths that appeared on her skin after local injures: pimples, scratches, cuts, and tattoos. She admits that her mother and sister have similar growths. She is anxious to have them removed. On exam there are multiple raised nodules with rounded, well-defined borders on her right shoulder and chest. Upon palpation they are slightly tender and have a rubber-like texture. Which of the following is/are true regarding her diagnosis?

A. Excision has a high risk of keloid recurrence.
B. Hispanic and African American populations have a higher rate of keloid occurrence.
C. Injections of corticosteroids and cryosurgery can diminish keloids.
D. The key to prevention is avoidance of any disruption of the skin.
E. All of the above

39. The answer is A: Cryosurgery. This patient has keloid formation at the site of her ear piercing. It is not uncommon for keloids to develop during pregnancy. Keloids are more common in dark-skinned races and represent excessive and dysregulated collagen deposition at the site of injury. Simple surgical treatment is often very difficult because keloids tend to recur and may get worse. Injections of glucocorticoids have shown some promise in shrinking lesions and relieving symptoms. Cryosurgery with repeated freezing over the course of a month has produced flattening of many lesions, but it is not always successful (**A**). Biopsy should not be performed, because it can exacerbate the keloid formation.

40. The answer is E: All of the above. Keloids are benign overgrowths of connective tissue arising from sites of dermal injury. They grow well beyond the dermal borders of injury, as opposed to a hypertrophic scar which remains within the borders of normal skin, and can be expected to grow over time. Because they are generated from trauma to the skin, keloid excision can lead to recurrence. Although periodic injections of triamcinolone and cryotherapy have both been used to diminish keloid size, ridding a patient of keloids is inherently difficult. Prevention is the key and educating patients about avoiding cosmetic or elective procedures such as piercings, tattoos, and plastic surgery is important. Darkly-pigmented populations have a higher incidence of keloids. Keloid proneness can also have a recessive or dominant pattern of familial inheritance (**E**).

Keloid

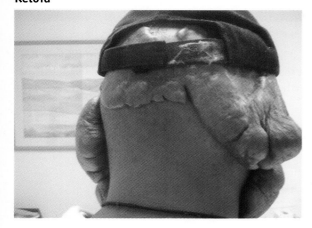

A *keloid* results from the uncontrolled synthesis and excessive deposition of collagen at sites of previous dermal injury and wound repair. They can occur after local skin trauma or inflammatory skin reactions. A keloid extends beyond the border of the original wound and resembles a well-circumscribed pink to purple nodule or pseudotumor. It does not regress spontaneously.

■ Dysregulated collagen deposition at site of dermal injury
■ Tend to recur after excision; difficult to treat
■ Predilection for areas of increased tension
■ More common in Asians and dark-skinned peoples

Notes

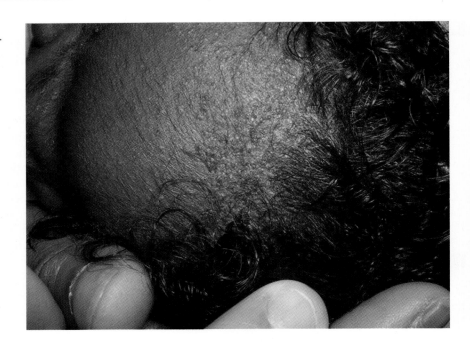

41. A 12-week-old infant is brought to the pediatrician with multiple yellow, greasy, flaky lesions over his scalp, especially along his hairline. His mother has tried several home remedies, but nothing has seemed to help. What therapy would you recommend?

A. Selenium sulfide shampoo
B. Oral fluconazole
C. Topical nystatin
D. Topical ketoconazole
E. Moisturizing lotion

42. A 43-year-old woman with a history of AIDS presents with dandruff and erythema and scaling of her eyebrows and nasolabial folds. You suspect seborrheic dermatitis. Which of the following treatments should be avoided in treating the facial scaling?

A. Antidandruff shampoo
B. Salicylic acid
C. Ketoconazole shampoo
D. Hydrocortisone cream
E. High-potency topical corticosteroids

41. **The answer is A: Selenium sulfide shampoo.** This infant has classic findings of seborrheic dermatitis, thought to be caused by overgrowth of the yeast, *Malassezia furfur*. Seborrheic dermatitis on the scalp responds to shampoos, such as selenium sulfide (**A**). Topical antifungals, such as ketoconazole (**D**), can be tried when the lesions are in other sebum-rich areas, but shampoos are used when lesions are present on the scalp. Topical nystatin (**C**) is often used to treat candida infections. Oral fluconazole (**B**) and other oral medications can be tried for refractive disease, but would not be the first-line choice, especially in a 12-week-old infant. Moisturizing lotion (**E**) will not provide any relief, because the affected areas are not caused by breaks in the skin due to dryness.

42. **The answer is E: High-potency topical corticosteroids.** Antidandruff shampoo (**A**), salicylic acid (**B**), ketoconazole (**C**) and hydrocortisone cream (**D**) are all appropriate options for treating seborrheic dermatitis. The use of higher potency topical corticosteroids (**E**) should be avoided on the face, as they can lead to steroid rosacea or perioral dermatitis.

Seborrheic Dermatitis

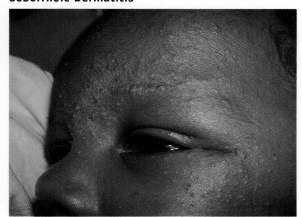

Seborrheic dermatitis, sometimes referred to as *cradle cap* when it occurs during infancy, is a skin disorder that can affect the scalp, face, or trunk. Skin appears greasy, yellow-red, flaky, and scaly. Seborrheic dermatitis particularly affects the sebum gland–rich areas of skin. The yeast, *Malassezia furfur,* is involved. Temporary hair loss may be a side effect to the inflammatory process. Topical treatments such as shampoos and creams are used in treatment.

- Greasy, yellow-red, flaky, scaly
- Usually nonpruritic
- Affects sebum-rich areas of skin
- Antifungals, such as ketoconazole, may be helpful in treatment.
- Outbreaks are usually worse in the winter and can be worsened by stress or fatigue.

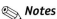 *Notes* _____

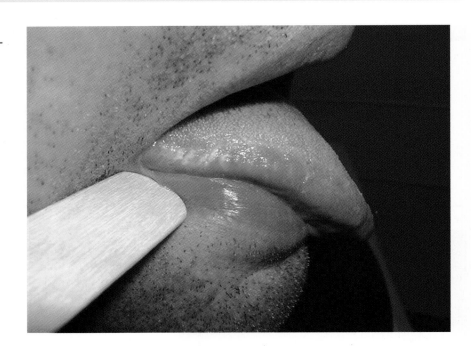

43. A 34-year-old man comes to the clinic to follow up on his antiretroviral therapy (ART). Six months ago, his CD4+ count was > 500/μL and viral load was < 10,000 copies of human immunodeficiency virus (HIV) RNA/mL. He has no complaints, but a new white, corrugated plaque is noted on the lateral aspect of his tongue on physical examination. It does not scrape off with a tongue blade. What is the next best step in this patient's treatment?

A. Punch biopsy and referral to otolaryngology or oral surgery for possible resection
B. Repeat CD4+ count, viral load, and perform drug-resistance testing
C. Oral fluconazole for 10-14 days
D. Cessation of ART
E. No action required

44. A 35-year-old African American man comes to clinic for his yearly physical. The patient has no complaints. He reports having had a flulike illness a few months ago. He was coughing with high fevers and chills in bed for more than 2 weeks. His social history is significant for multiple male and female sexual partners with intermittent condom use. On physical exam there is anterior and posterior cervical lymphadenopathy, as well as a 1-cm white, adherent, corrugated, nontender patch on the left anterolateral lingual margin. A clinical diagnosis of oral hairy leukoplakia (OHL) is made. The patient is positive for HIV on initial ELISA test and confirmed with a Western blot. Which of the following is/are true regarding OHL?

A. It represents a local Epstein-Barr virus (EBV) infection
B. Seen only in immunocompromised states
C. Treatment is directed at underlying condition
D. It is a benign lesion
E. All of the above

43. The answer is B: Repeat CD4+ count, viral load, and perform drug-resistance testing. This patient has OHL, which is a benign lesion of the oral mucosa representing EBV infection. It most often appears as an asymptomatic, corrugated white plaque on the inferolateral aspects of the tongue and does not scrape off. While the lesion itself does not need treatment, it may herald the failure of ART or the development of drug resistance. Candida coinfection can be present, but it will scrape off, as opposed to OHL. The appearance of OHL carries poor prognosis in HIV disease and demands retesting of CD4+ counts, viral load, and investigation into resistance (**B**).

44. The answer is E: All of the above. OHL remains an important clinical sign of underlying immunosuppression (HIV, organ transplant, extended steroid use, chemotherapy). As in this case, OHL can be the herald of HIV infection. This clinical picture prompted HIV testing. Even though patients with OHL and HIV are at higher risk of developing malignancies (lymphoma), OHL is itself a benign lesion that is rarely symptomatic. It appears on the lateral borders of the tongue as a fixed, white or gray, corrugated patch that may not be removed by scraping. EBV replicates freely within the lesion, where candida infection may coexist. The lesion will resolve with highly active antiretroviral therapy (HAART) and subsequent restoration of immunocompetence (**E**).

Hairy Leukoplakia

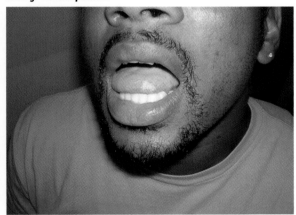

Oral hairy leukoplakia (OHL) is a benign hyperplasia of the oral mucosa that most frequently appears on the lateral or inferior aspect of the tongue. It represents EBV infection and presents as asymptomatic, corrugated white plaques with accentuation of the vertical folds. It is seen primarily in the HIV population.

- EBV infection in the HIV population; candida coinfection may be present
- Not a premalignant condition, but associated with poorer prognosis in HIV disease
- Lesion regresses or clears with HAART; development may herald failure of HAART or the development of drug-resistance

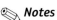

✎ *Notes*
_____

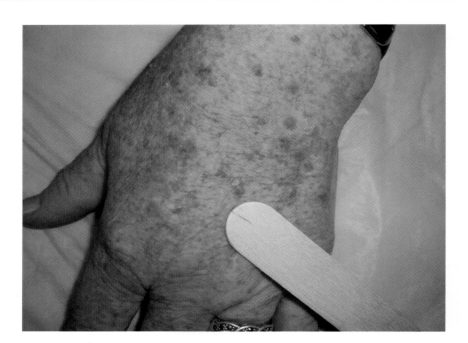

45. A 67-year-old Caucasian man comes to the office for the first time. He recently moved to the area and works part time on a fishing boat. He previously worked as a landscaper and trash collector. He has no complaints, although his past medical history is significant for a skin biopsy on his shoulder "for a dark mole" 10 years ago. As he speaks, his hands are visible (shown above). Similar lesions are present on his cheeks and temples. The lesions are rough and scaly and range from 1-5 mm in diameter. What is the next best step for the lesions on his hand?

A. Reassurance with no further workup
B. Biopsy
C. Cryosurgery
D. Recommend UVA/UVB sunscreen with no further workup
E. Wide local excision

46. A 62-year-old farmer is concerned about a rough patch on his lip. It has been there for more than a year and has not changed during this time. It is not painful. He has had similar lesions on his hands and the top of his head, some of which have been "frozen" by his dermatologist. On examination, the lesion appears well-demarcated and has an ulcerated base. What is the next best step in management?

A. Reassurance with no further workup
B. Biopsy
C. Cryosurgery
D. Recommend UVA/UVB sunscreen with no further workup
E. Wide local excision

45. **The answer is C: Cryosurgery.** The patient's history of sun exposure, combined with the appearance and description (rough and scaly) of the lesions, makes actinic keratosis the likely diagnosis. Since actinic keratosis can progress to squamous cell carcinoma, the lesions should be treated. Cryosurgery works in most cases (**C**). Actinic keratosis can usually be diagnosed clinically; however, highly hyperkeratotic lesions, as well as those that are painful, bleeding, ulcerated, or rapidly growing, should be biopsied to rule out malignancy (**B**). Sunscreen is an important preventive measure (**D**), but treatment is warranted at this time. Wide local excision is the treatment if squamous cell carcinoma is diagnosed (**E**).

46. **The answer is B: Biopsy.** The lesion most likely represents actinic keratosis. It is a well-demarcated, stable lesion in an exposed area on a light-skinned man who has worked extensively outdoors. However, actinic keratosis can progress to squamous cell carcinoma, and ulceration is a concerning feature. Thus biopsy is warranted (**B**). His history is suggestive of cryosurgery (**C**) for other lesions, and this may be an appropriate treatment in this case if the biopsy is negative. Sunscreen (**D**) should be recommended as a preventive measure but does not resolve the question of how to manage the current lesion. Because this is likely actinic keratosis, wide local excision (**E**) is not appropriate at this time.

Actinic Keratosis

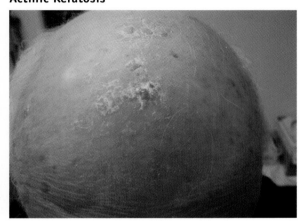

Actinic keratosis consists of rough, adherent, scaly lesions that are often erythematous and painful when scratched. They result from proliferation of abnormal epidermal keratinocytes in response to prolonged UV radiation exposure.

- Precursor of squamous cell carcinoma
- The most important risk factor is exposure to sunlight. Look for an older, light-skinned individual who has spent a lot of time outdoors.
- Diagnose clinically. Highly hyperkeratotic lesions may need biopsy to rule out squamous cell carcinoma.
- It should be treated to prevent progression to squamous cell carcinoma. Options include cryosurgery, topical agents, curettage, and phototherapy.

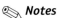 *Notes*

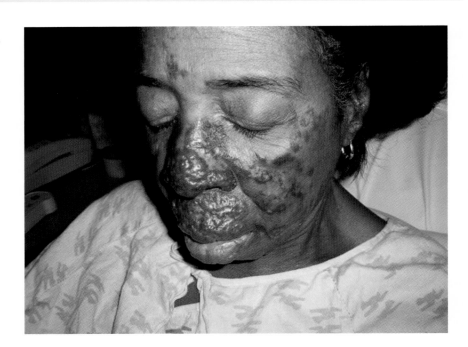

47. A 63-year-old African American woman presents with a large violaceous plaque over the bridge of her nose, her cheeks, and her upper lip. She also complains of cough and dyspnea. A chest x-ray reveals bilateral hilar adenopathy. Which of the following findings would you expect?

A. Biopsy of the skin lesion showing noncaseating granuloma
B. Biopsy of the lung showing caseating granuloma
C. Low serum angiotensin-converting enzyme (ACE) level
D. Pulmonary function test (PFT) showing obstructive pattern
E. Positive rapid plasma reagin (RPR)

48. A 34-year-old African American man presents with worsening shortness of breath, chest pain, and cough of 3 months' duration. He also complains of fatigue and general malaise, describing a 10-pound weight loss over the last 3 months. This is the first time he has experienced symptoms like this, and he denies any history of travel or incarceration. He works as a librarian and denies alcohol, drug, or tobacco use. Physical exam reveals patchy crackles. Chest x-ray shows mediastinal adenopathy, and biopsy of one of the lesions reveals noncaseating granulomas. His HIV test is negative. Which of the following is the most appropriate initial treatment for this patient?

A. INH and rifampin
B. Chemotherapy
C. Cyclophosphamide
D. Glucocorticoids
E. Infliximab

47. The answer is A: Biopsy of the skin lesion showing noncaseating granuloma. The violaceous plaque over this woman's face is lupus pernio, which is a cutaneous manifestation of sarcoidosis. This woman also has bilateral hilar adenopathy, a classic finding in sarcoidosis, which indicates lung involvement. A biopsy of the lung or skin lesion would show noncaseating granulomas (**A**). Caseating granulomas on lung biopsy (**B**) are suggestive of tuberculosis (TB). Up to 75% of untreated sarcoid patients will have an elevated ACE level, thus a low serum ACE level (**C**) would not aid in making a diagnosis. When lung involvement is present in sarcoidosis, a restrictive pattern is seen on PFTs rather than an obstructive pattern (**D**). RPR (**E**) is a screening test for syphilis.

48. The answer is D: Glucocorticoids. This patient is suffering from sarcoidosis, a multisystem disease that most frequently involves the lungs. Other manifestations include erythema nodosum, acute polyarthritis, and anterior uveitis. Mediastinal and paratracheal adenopathy are highly suggestive of sarcoidosis. Additional classic findings on chest X-ray include reticulonodular infiltrates and biopsy will demonstrate noncaseating granulomas. Asymptomatic sarcoidosis is often followed closely without treatment due to the high rate of spontaneous remission, but patients with symptomatic disease receive systemic glucocorticoids (**D**) as initial treatment for sarcoidosis. INH and rifampin (**A**) are part of the typical four drug regimen used to treat active TB. While TB could explain many of this patient's symptoms, biopsy would show caseating granulomas. Cyclophosphamide (**C**) is a chemotherapeutic agent that is often used to treat systemic lupus erythematosus with renal involvement and is not an appropriate initial treatment for sarcoidosis. Infliximab is a tumor necrosis–alpha inhibitor (TNF-alpha inhibitor) approved for the use in ankylosing spondylitis, inflammatory bowel disease, and rheumatoid arthritis. Neither infliximab nor chemotherapy (**B**) would be an appropriate treatment for this patient.

Sarcoidosis (Noncaseating Granulomas)

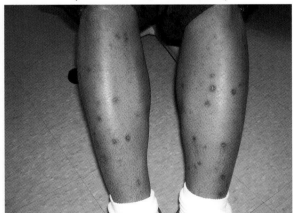

Sarcoidosis is a systemic granulomatous inflammatory disease of unknown etiology. The disease is characterized by noncaseating granulomas. Granulomas are most often noted in the lungs or lymph nodes, but almost any organ can be affected. The highest incidence is in Northern American blacks and Northern European whites. Among blacks, women are more frequently affected than men.

Disease onset is usually in the 30s or 40s. Lupus pernio is a severe cutaneous manifestation of sarcoidosis. Violaceous plaques can occur on the nose, cheeks, ears, lips, and fingers. Diagnosis of sarcoidosis requires three components: clinical and radiographic manifestations, exclusion of other diseases with similar presentations, and the presence of noncaseating granulomas. Chest x-ray, pulmonary function tests, ECG, slit-lamp eye exam, liver function tests, and serum calcium test should be included in the initial evaluation of a patient with suspected sarcoidosis. Glucocorticoids are the initial treatment.

- Bilateral hilar adenopathy may be seen on imaging.
- Treat with corticosteroids. Other immunosuppressive drugs, cyclosporine, and anti-TNF therapy with infliximab have also been used.
- Pulmonary function tests characteristically reveal a restrictive pattern if there is lung involvement.
- Elevated serum ACE level in 75% of untreated patients
- Histopathologic detection of noncaseating granuloma is helpful to make diagnosis.
- Common presenting symptoms include cough, dyspnea, chest pain, eye lesions, and/or skin lesions.

Notes _____

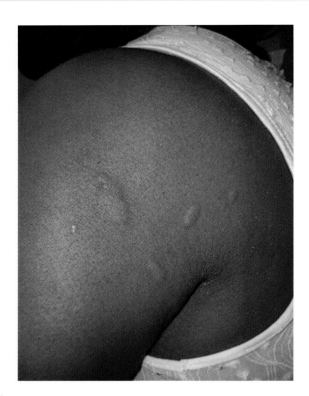

49. A 23-year-old man presents with pruritic lesions on his right arm which appeared about 24 hours ago over his upper arm. The lesions appear as central rounded localized areas of edema with peripheral erythema. How would you define the central area of edema?

A. Flare
B. Wheal
C. Vesicle
D. Bulla
E. Cyst

50. A 45-year-old woman comes to your office complaining of a raised, red, itchy lesion with a central area of edema and peripheral erythema that appeared a few hours after being bitten by a mosquito. She has a formal event tomorrow and is concerned about how long this unsightly mark will remain on her arm. What is the best advice for this patient?

A. This lesion will likely fade in 7 days.
B. This lesion will likely progress to a disseminated rash in 3-7 days.
C. This lesion will likely go away in 24-48 hours.
D. Corticosteroids are necessary for the treatment of this lesion.
E. Biopsy is warranted for definitive diagnosis.

49. **The answer is B: Wheal.** This patient has urticaria (hives), which typically last 24-48 hours. The lesions are pruritic and classically demonstrate a central wheal (**B**). The wheal is the area of localized edema. Surrounding the wheal, a flat area of erythema is often present, referred to as the *flare* (**A**). Although the lesion is similar to a vesicle (**C**), a small, fluid-filled, elevated lesion, the evanescent nature of the lesion and the associated pruritic description indicate urticaria. A bulla (**D**) is a large vesicle. A cyst (**E**) is an epithelial-lined sac containing fluid or semisolid material.

50. **The answer is C: This lesion will likely go away in 24-48 hours.** This patient is experiencing an allergic reaction from the insect bite known as a wheal and flare reaction that will likely resolve in 24-48 hours without any treatment (**C**). Corticosteroids are not necessary for the treatment of this lesion (**D**). Clinical diagnosis suffices in this case, and biopsy is not warranted unless the lesion persists (**E**).

Wheal

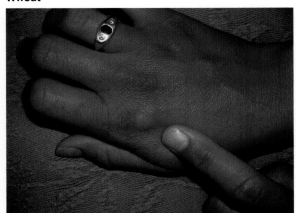

A *wheal* is a primary skin lesion and is defined as a rounded or flat-topped, pale-red papule or plaque that is typically evanescent, disappearing within 24-48 hours. A wheal appears as an area of localized edema that follows vascular leakage. A wheal and flare skin reaction is often associated with an allergic reaction. The wheal is the central raised area, which is surrounded by a flat erythematous flare.

- Typically last 24-48 hours
- Primary skin lesion
- Localized edema

Notes _____

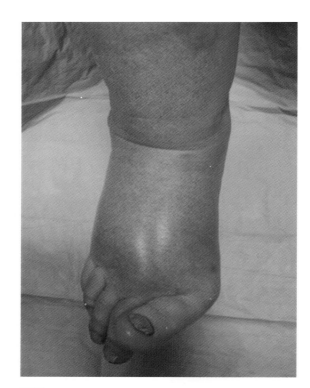

51. A 56-year-old woman comes to the office for a postoperative visit 1 week after open-fixation of an ankle fracture and complains of pain and swelling in her foot (pictured above). She states that she first noticed a patch of redness and some pain near the surgical incision last night but woke up to find it had spread to encompass her entire foot. She reports that she "just doesn't feel well," and reports chills overnight. On physical exam, her temperature is 101° F (38.3° C), blood pressure 118/78, and heart rate 86 beats per minute (bpm). The right foot is edematous, erythematous, warm, and tender to the touch with no crepitus or fluctuance present. The incision site is intact, and no purulent material is noted. Which of the following infectious organisms should be suspected in this patient?

A. Group A β-hemolytic streptococci
B. *Pseudomonas aeruginosa*
C. *Staphylococcus aureus*
D. *Escherichia coli* and other gram-negative species
E. All except B

52. A 77-year-old Caucasian woman was recently bitten on the hand by her housecat. The cat has been vaccinated against rabies and never leaves the house. The woman has a history of hypertension and hyperlipidemia but is otherwise healthy. Her hand is erythematous and edematous. Strength in her fingers and wrist is 5/5. An x-ray showed no tooth fragments or bony injury. Cultures are pending. She is given tetanus toxoid in the ED. Which of the following is the best treatment?

A. Amoxicillin-clavulanate
B. Cefepime
C. Ciprofloxacin
D. Clindamycin
E. No treatment necessary

51. **The answer is E: All except B.** This patient has cellulitis that she developed after a surgical procedure. The defect in the skin barrier and any metal hardware installed during the procedure are risks for developing this type of infection. She has the classic findings of edema, erythema, warmth, and pain. The lack of crepitus and fluctuance is reassuring that this infection is not necrotizing fasciitis or an abscess. Common pathogens for cellulitis include group A β-hemolytic streptococci and *S. aureus* species; however, this patient is also at risk for *E. coli* and gram-negative infection because the wound is below the waist. Thus initial antibiotic coverage should have activity against these pathogens and can be adjusted later if the pathogen(s) can be identified (**E**).

52. **The answer is A: Amoxicillin-clavulanate.** The patient has cellulitis from a cat bite and is likely infected with *Pasteurella multocida*. The best antibiotic choice is oral amoxicillin/clavulanic acid for 7-10 days (**A**). Alternatives include oral doxycycline or clindamycin plus a fluoroquinolone. Clindamycin alone and cephalosporins do not provide coverage against *P. multicida* (**B, C, D**). Cat bites often penetrate to tendons and bones. The wound should be examined for depth of injury and possible joint penetration. Nerve and tendon function and integrity of nearby vessels should be determined, and an x-ray should be obtained to exclude retained tooth fragments, fracture, and/or crush injury, which may occur in the setting of an animal bite.

Cellulitis

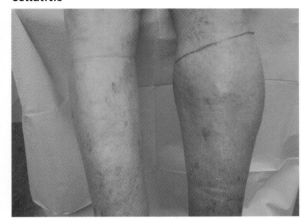

Cellulitis is an acute inflammatory reaction representing a spreading infection of the dermis and subcutaneous tissue. The most common pathogens include group A β-hemolytic streptococci and *S. aureus*. It typically presents as a small patch of swelling, erythema, and pain before spreading diffusely. As the infection spreads, the patient may experience fever, chills, and malaise, and is at risk for developing septicemia.

- Edematous, expanding, erythematous, warm plaque with ill-defined borders
- Pathogens gain entry to dermis and subcutaneous tissue through defects in the skin barrier, including cuts, cracks, abrasions, burns, insect bites, surgical incisions, or foreign bodies such as IV catheters.
- Biopsy and aspiration of the leading edge have low yield in identifying the pathogen. Blood cultures or culture from an ulcer, pustule, or abscess, if present, may be useful.

Notes

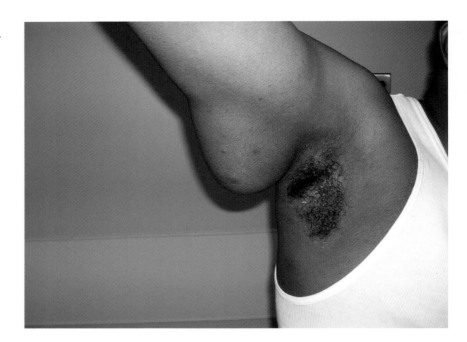

53. A 35-year-old man notices a slow growing mass on his arm. The mass is mildly tender, and he is concerned because the mass is large and noticeable to others. Physical examination reveals a rubbery, soft, fluctuant mass with lobulation and free mobility of the overlying skin. What is the most likely diagnosis?

A. Lymphoma
B. Liposarcoma
C. Lipoma
D. Glomus tumor
E. Cutaneous leiomyoma

54. A 50-year-old man presents to his primary care physician with a large mass on his upper back. The mass is painless and, aside from being uncomfortable due to its size, has not otherwise affected the patient. He is, however, concerned that he might have cancer because the mass has been slowly growing over the past 5 years. On physical exam the mass is superficial, nontender, homogeneous, and rubbery. Although the physician feels the mass is highly likely to be benign, a biopsy is conducted to better characterize the tissue and assure the patient. What is the most likely histological finding?

A. A mixture of mature adipocytes and a chondroid matrix containing lipoblasts.
B. Unencapsulated bundles of pleomorphic spindle cells and multinucleate giant cells mixed with lipoblasts.
C. Large numbers of brown fat cells mixed with mature white fat.
D. Lobules of mature white adipose tissue divided by fibrous septa containing thin-walled, capillary-sized vessels.
E. A proliferation of adipose and fibrous tissue within the epineurium infiltrating along and between nerve bundles.

53. **The answer is C: Lipoma.** Superficial subcutaneous lipomas are common, benign neoplasms of the skin. They rarely cause symptoms, but patients often bring them to the attention of their providers either because they are either worried about the possibility of cancer or because of the cosmetic deformity caused by larger lesions. Clinical history is used to distinguish lipoma from more serious conditions such as lymphoma (**A**) based on the fact that lipomas are soft, asymptomatic, and usually do not enlarge quickly. Malignant transformation of a lipoma into a liposarcoma (**B**) is rare. Liposarcomas typically appear in the deep fat tissue of the thigh or abdomen in people between the ages of 50 and 70. If a suspected lipoma causes symptoms, is rapidly enlarging, or is firm rather than soft, a biopsy is indicated. Glomus tumors (**D**) are small benign tumors that arise from the glomus body. Cutaneous leiomyomas (**E**) are benign soft tissue neoplasms that arise from the smooth muscle and may involve vascular smooth muscle, the dartos muscles of the genitalia, the nipples, or the areolas.

54. **The answer is D: Lobules of mature white adipose tissue divided by fibrous septa containing thin-walled, capillary-sized vessels.** This patient is presenting with a lipoma (**D**), the most common soft-tissue neoplasm. These tumors occur predominantly in individuals between 40 and 60 years old, but may affect patients in a wide age range. Lipomas are entirely benign mesenchymal neoplasms. The most common presentation is as a painless subcutaneous mass typically occurring on the trunk, neck, or extremities.

Less commonly, lipomas may be found deep in the subcutaneous tissue or intramuscularly and may be painful to patients. Histologically these tumors are circumscribed, encapsulated by a thin, fibrous capsule, and composed of mature white adipocytes lacking evidence of nuclear atypia. Because lipomas are entirely benign, they may be left alone without concern for malignant potential unless they cause discomfort to a patient. In the instance of very large tumors or intramuscular lipomas, surgical excision is the treatment of choice. (**A**) Chondroid lipomas are rare benign tumors occurring most commonly in adult women and tend to be smaller than 5 cm. They are characterized histologically by an admixture of a mature adipocytic component and a chondroid matrix containing lipoblasts. (**B**) Pleomorphic liposarcomas are aggressive sarcomas found on the extremities of adults and are associated with high rates of metastasis and mortality. These deep-seated tumors tend to grow rapidly and are less frequently found in subcutaneous tissue. Histologically they are characterized by features of a high-grade pleomorphic sarcoma containing spindle cells and multinucleated giant cells with admixed lipoblasts. (**C**) Hibernomas are rare benign neoplasms containing brown fat. They most commonly affect young adults and are most frequently found in the thigh region. (**E**) Lipomatosis of nerve is a rare tumor that affects infants and children and presents as a growing mass, most commonly on the hand. Histologically, lesions are characterized by a proliferation of adipose and fibrous tissue within the epineurium, infiltrating along and in between nerve bundles.

Lipoma

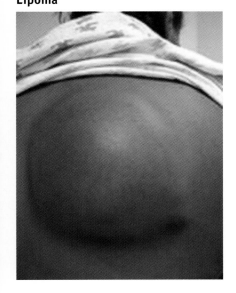

A *lipoma* is a benign tumor of mature fat cells enclosed by a thin, fibrous capsule. They are most often found superficially in the subcutaneous tissue but can more rarely involve fascia or deeper muscular planes.

- Familial multiple lipomatosis is a genetic condition resulting in multiple lipomas.
- Diagnostic workup: CT or ultrasound (not MRI), excision, biopsy
- Surgical removal of the fat cells and fibrous capsule is indicated for cosmetic reasons if the lipoma causes pain, or for tissue to confirm diagnosis.

Notes

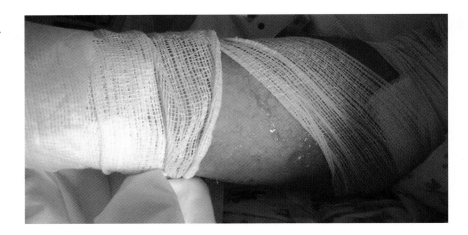

55. A previously healthy 64-year-old man presents with localized pain, erythema, and swelling surrounding a small wound on his right hand. These symptoms rapidly progressed to involve his entire right arm, and his pain became severe. He also developed fever and diarrhea. Initial laboratory evaluation reveals an elevated WBC and an elevated creatine phosphokinase. In addition to empiric antibiotics, what would be the next step in treatment?

A. Reexamine patient in 24 hours
B. Ultrasound of right arm
C. Send patient for immediate MRI
D. Culture wound on patient's right hand
E. Surgical exploration and debridement

56. A 61-year-old man with a past medical history of type 2 diabetes mellitus, IV drug use, and chronic skin infections presents to the ED with a 3-day history of subjective fever and confusion along with swelling, redness, and blisters on his right arm. The patient admits that he had been "skin-popping" IV heroin in his right arm in the week prior to the onset of his symptoms. Physical exam reveals erythema, brawny edema, and severe pain with very minimal passive movement of the right extremity. There are several large bullae seen on his right forearm, along with crepitus in the overlying skin. What is most important first step in the management of this patient's condition?

A. MRI of the right upper extremity
B. Surgical consult
C. Transfusion of two units of packed red blood cells
D. Lance of the bullae and culture fluid
E. Hyperbaric oxygen therapy

55. **The answer is E: Surgical exploration and debridement.** This patient is presenting with findings that are concerning for necrotizing fasciitis. This is a surgical emergency and requires exploration and debridement (**E**). Surgical exploration is the only way to confirm the diagnosis, and prompt surgical exploration facilitates early debridement. Broad-spectrum IV antibiotics should be administered. Reexamining the patient in 24 hours (**A**) is not appropriate, given the likelihood of rapid progression. Although necrotizing fasciitis must be distinguished from other processes, such as gas gangrene, pyomyositis, and myositis, the history and clinical features usually allow this distinction. Laboratory findings are not specific. Imaging may be useful in some instances. CT is most commonly used to visualize air along the fascial planes. MRI and ultrasound (**B, C**) may not delineate air along the fascial planes. MRI often cannot distinguish necrotizing fasciitis from cellulitis or inflammation. Gram stain and culture of the lesion (**D**) may be positive for organisms, but this is not as reliable as obtaining deep samples during surgical exploration. If the diagnosis of necrotizing fasciitis is suspected, awaiting the results of blood or skin cultures is not recommended.

56. **The answer is B: Surgical consult.** This patient presents with the classic symptoms of a necrotizing soft tissue infection, which include tissue pain out of proportion to physical examination findings, erythema, brawny edema, and crepitus. Bullae develop later in the course of the infection. This patient has several risk factors for a necrotizing soft tissue infection, including diabetes mellitus, advanced age, chronic skin infections, and IV drug abuse. Several other risk factors are alcoholism, peripheral vascular disease, heart disease, renal failure, HIV, cancer, NSAID use, decubitus ulcers, and immune system impairment. Necrotizing fasciitis is a clinical diagnosis based on physical exam findings and patient history. This patient's past medical history, especially his IV drug use, make the diagnosis highly likely. Necrotizing soft tissue infections are a surgical emergency, and early surgical consultation (**B**) is the most important first step in the management of all suspected cases of necrotizing fasciitis, and the gold standard for diagnosis and therapy remains operative exploration and surgical debridement. MRI (**A**) is highly sensitive in identifying fascial thickening and deep tissue collections but delays definitive surgical treatment. Blood transfusion (**C**) may be indicated later to correct anemia from hemolysis but is not the first step in management. Although cultures of blood and bullae fluid (**D**) may be helpful later in the treatment when antibiotic coverage is narrowed, it is more important to get the patient into the operating room for exploration and debridement. Hyperbaric oxygen therapy (**E**) is a controversial therapy that would be the decision of the surgical consult and would not be part of the initial treatment of a patient in the ED.

Necrotizing Fasciitis

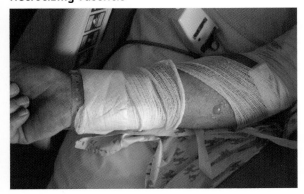

Necrotizing fasciitis is an infection of the deep layers of skin and subcutaneous tissue that easily spreads across the fascial planes. Necrotizing fasciitis may present initially with localized pain, erythema, and swelling. However, rapid progression may follow, resulting in bullae formation and systemic symptoms. If untreated, the bacteria can travel rapidly along the fascia of the muscle and spread throughout the body, leading to sepsis and death. There are two types of necrotizing fasciitis. Type 1 is a mixed organismal infection that occurs postsurgically, often in patients with diabetes or peripheral vascular disease. Type 2 is a monomicrobial infection caused principally by group A streptococcus (*Streptococcus pyogenes*).

- If there is clinical suspicion of necrotizing fasciitis, surgical exploration should be done for definitive diagnosis. No lab tests can rapidly and accurately differentiate between necrotizing fasciitis and other soft tissue infections.
- Treat with multiple episodes of surgical debridement, hemodynamic support, and empiric IV antibiotics.
- *Streptococcus pyogenes* releases an exotoxin known as *superantigen* which activates T cells and leads to the overproduction of cytokines.

Notes

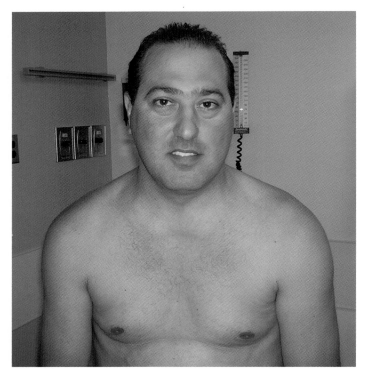

57. A 36-year-old man comes to the clinic complaining of weakness. He states he has recently noticed a lack of energy and frequently experiences backaches and headaches. He is also concerned about recent changes in his appearance. Examination reveals plethoric moon facies, supraclavicular fat pads, and a protuberant abdomen. He does not smoke or drink alcohol and takes no medications. Past medical history is significant only for cellulitis 2 months prior. Which sequence of tests would confirm the diagnosis?

A. Serum adrenocorticotropic hormone (ACTH) level and MRI of the head
B. Dexamethasone suppression test, urine free cortisol, and serum ACTH
C. CT scan of the chest and abdomen
D. Midnight serum cortisol, morning serum cortisol, and random serum cortisol tests
E. No further testing necessary

58. A 22-year-old woman comes to the clinic because she is concerned about changes in her appearance, as well as decreased libido and irregular menses, which she reports have been worsening over the past several years. She feels that her face has gotten larger, and she no longer feels attractive. She also reports that her skin has become dark spotted, and she has noticed purple lines on her abdomen. In the last few months, she has given up on physical activity because she feels weak. Examination reveals plethoric moon facies, supraclavicular fat pads, and central obesity. Her blood pressure is 150/90. She does not smoke or drink alcohol. She takes no medications. Past medical history is significant only for recurrent infections in recent years. Which of the following describe changes seen in the most likely diagnosis of this patient?

A. Increase in serum ACTH level produced by the anterior pituitary
B. Increase in cortisol level and decrease of ACTH level
C. Increase in ACTH level produced ectopically
D. Decrease in cortisol level due to adrenal insufficiency
E. Electrolyte disturbances, normal ACTH levels

57. The answer is B: Dexamethasone suppression test, urine free cortisol, and serum ACTH. This patient displays the physical and symptomatic manifestations of hypercortisolism in Cushing syndrome, and his condition warrants a workup (**E**). The correct sequence of confirmatory laboratory testing is a dexamethasone suppression test, urine free cortisol, and serum ACTH (**B**). Dexamethasone suppression testing is performed by giving 1 mg of dexamethasone orally at 11 PM and assessing serum cortisol at 8 AM the following morning. An abnormal test result warrants confirmation of excess cortisol by 24-hour urine free cortisol testing, midnight cortisol levels, or a late-night salivary cortisol assay (**D**). Once hypercortisolism is established, serum ACTH levels should be assessed. A level of ACTH below 20 pg/mL indicates a probable adrenal tumor, whereas higher levels are the result of a pituitary tumor (termed *Cushing disease*) or ectopic ACTH production. Imaging techniques for localization of the lesion are indicated once the initial workup has been completed (**A, C**).

58. The answer is A: Increase in serum ACTH level produced by the anterior pituitary. The patient suffers from Cushing syndrome (**A**), due to increased production of ACTH. She has typical signs of this disorder, including round plethoric facies, purple skin striae, and central obesity. She also has symptoms of weakness, menstrual irregularities, and sexual dysfunction. Cortisol increases secondary to an increase in ACTH, rather than a decrease (**B**). The patient is not a smoker, so the increased in ACTH is not likely due to ectopic production from a malignant tumor, such as small cell carcinoma of the lung (**C**). Addison disease causes an increase in ACTH (because of lack of negative feedback). Typically it presents as an increase in skin pigmentation but is not associated with the other symptoms seen in this case (**D**). Conn syndrome results in electrolyte disturbances and muscle weakness, but the other symptoms in this case are not explained by this disease (**E**).

Cushing Syndrome

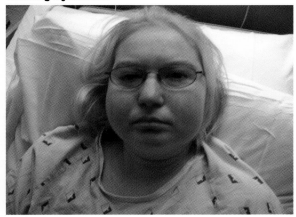

Cushing syndrome refers to the state of excess corticosteroids and the resultant physical manifestations. The most frequent cause is iatrogenic. Cushing syndrome is less frequently due to endogenous excess corticosteroid production by the adrenal cortex. Cushing disease accounts for nearly 40% of cases and describes the scenario where the manifestations of excess corticosteroids result from the hypersecretion of ACTH by a benign pituitary adenoma, most frequently located in the anterior pituitary. Occasionally, hypercortisolism may represent a paraneoplastic condition where nonpituitary neoplasms like small cell lung cancer produce and secrete ACTH. Excess corticosteroid production independent of ACTH is due to autonomous secretion of cortisol by the adrenals, usually from a unilateral adrenal tumor.

- Central obesity, moon facies, protuberant abdomen, muscle wasting, thin skin, hirsutism, purple striae, buffalo hump, supraclavicular fat pads
- Osteoporosis, hypertension, poor wound healing, easy bruising, superficial skin infections, and susceptibility to opportunistic infections
- Women: oligomenorrhea or amenorrhea; males: impotence
- Psychologic changes: decreased concentration, mood liability, frank psychosis
- Hyperglycemia, glycosuria, leukocytosis, lymphocytopenia, hypokalemia
- Elevated serum cortisol and urine free cortisol; lack of normal suppression by dexamethasone

Notes

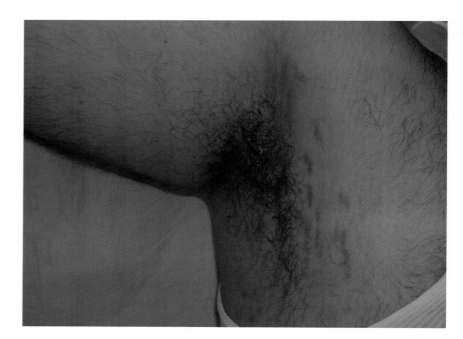

59. A 41-year-old male patient has been on long-term high-dose steroids for Crohn disease. He is concerned because he has noticed an increasing number of well-defined, symmetric, elevated, reddish-purple lesions in his axilla. He also has several older lesions which have faded to a pale color. Which of the following options may help to improve the appearance of these lesions?

A. Topical tretinoin
B. Glycolic acid cream
C. Stop high-dose steroid treatment
D. Laser surgery
E. All of the above

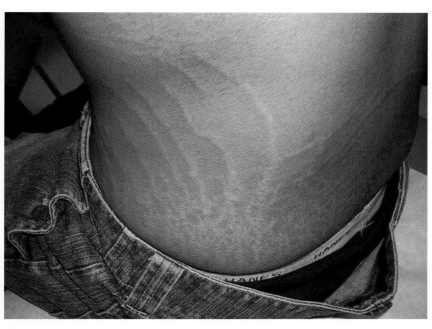

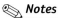 *Notes*

60. A 28-year-old woman with a history of severe asthma presents to your office complaining of recent weight gain. She is frustrated after trying many diets and comes to you for advice. Upon further questioning, the patient also describes stretch marks on her abdomen and fatty growth on her neck and shoulders. You notice that her arms and legs are still quite thin and her face appears moonlike. She seems to be concealing her armpits which you notice to be quite sweaty. Which of the following is the best step in diagnosing her condition?

A. Glucose tolerance test
B. MRI of the pituitary gland
C. Fasting plasma glucose level
D. CT of the adrenal glands
E. Dexamethasone suppression test

59. The answer is E: All of the above. All of the above treatments (**E**) are known to help improve the progression of striae (stretch marks). Although the lesions are not reversible, there are treatments that can help to fade the lesions. Topical tretinoin (**A**), glycolic acid creams (**B**), and stopping steroid treatment (**C**) will help to fade striae. In addition, laser surgery (**D**) has been shown in some cases to improve the appearance of stretch marks.

60. The answer is E. The most common cause of Cushing syndrome is the exogenous administration of corticosteroids by a health care provider, in this case to treat this patient's severe asthma. The patient's symptoms, central obesity, striae, and hyperhidrosis, in the setting of likely steroid use, suggest exogenous Cushing syndrome. When Cushing syndrome is suspected, either a dexamethasone suppression test or a 24-hour urine cortisol measurement is indicated as the next step in diagnosis. If this test is positive, an MRI of the pituitary gland or CT of the adrenal gland may be performed to detect the presence of any adrenal or pituitary adenomas or incidentalomas (**B, D**). While this patient likely has impaired glucose tolerance due to Cushing syndrome, a glucose tolerance test (**A**) or fasting plasma glucose level (**C**) is not necessary at this time.

Striae

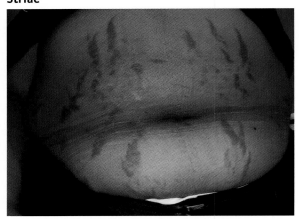

Striae, or stretch marks, are well-defined, symmetric, trophic lesions. They are caused by a tearing of the dermis and are a form of scarring that produces an off-color hue. They first appear as elevated reddish or purple lines in areas of rapid growth; however, they eventually flatten and fade to a pale color. Striae are often the result of rapid skin stretching. They may be associated with times of rapid growth such as puberty, weight gain, and pregnancy. In addition, striae formation is influenced by hormonal changes. Glucocorticoid hormones cause striae formation by preventing fibroblasts from forming collagen and elastin fibers necessary to keep rapidly growing skin taut. Thus striae may occur in patients with Cushing syndrome or in patients chronically treated with high-dose steroids. They can occur anywhere on the body but are most likely to appear in areas of larger fat stores (abdomen, breasts, upper arms, back, thighs, hips, buttocks). Striae are more common in women. Early-stage striae have shown improvement with the use of topical tretinoin and glycolic acid creams. Laser therapy has been shown in some cases to improve the appearance of striae as well.

- Tearing of the dermis
- Appear in areas with larger fat stores
- Associated with times of rapid growth
- Influenced by hormonal changes

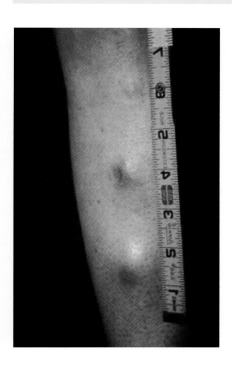

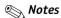

61. A 27-year-old woman presents to the clinic complaining of pain in her lower legs for the past 2 days. Over this time she has been feeling ill and also complains of bilateral ankle pain. On physical exam, her temperature is 100.4° F (38° C), and her blood pressure is 142/92. Erythematous lesions that are nodular and tender to palpation are seen on her lower legs (shown above). ESR and c-reactive protein are elevated. A chest radiograph reveals bilateral adenopathy, and sarcoidosis is suspected. The patient is scheduled for tissue biopsies. What is the best management of her lower limb findings at this time?

A. Topical corticosteroids
B. Oral prednisone with a taper
C. NSAIDs and symptomatic treatment
D. Bilateral ankle aspiration and radiographs
E. Biopsy of the edge of a nodule

62. A 23-year-old women presents to the clinic with pleuritic chest pain, bronchial cough, fatigue, and a fever for 2 weeks. She says that she went hiking and camping in southern Arizona 1 month ago. She thought she had picked up a bad cold. Her fever resolved 3 days ago; however, her fatigue, cough, and chest pain continue. She was prompted to come in yesterday when she noticed painful red nodules on her lower legs and aching knee pain. Physical exam is significant for right-sided crackles and 2- to 3-cm hard, red, tender nodules on the extensor surfaces of the lower legs. A chest x-ray shows a right middle lobe infiltrate and right hilar adenopathy. Sputum cultures are sent. Tissue samples obtained via bronchoscopy reveal spherules filled with endospores. What is the best management at this time?

A. Oral corticosteroids
B. Ampicillin-clavulanate
C. NSAIDs and symptomatic treatment
D. Fluconazole
E. C and D only

61. **The answer is C: NSAIDs and symptomatic treatment.** This patient has erythema nodosum and suspected sarcoidosis. Erythema nodosum is an immunologic skin reaction showing granulomatous inflammation that has a variety of causes, including drugs, infection, inflammatory or granulomatous disease, and malignancy. Treatment is symptomatic, antiinflammatory (**C**), and directed at the underlying cause if known. Patients often have associated fever, malaise, and arthralgia, particularly of the ankle joints. Glucocorticoids should be used only if the etiology is known. Women are affected 10 times more frequently than men. Lesions will typically disappear after 6 weeks but may recur.

62. **The answer is E: C and D only.** This patient has confirmed coccidioidomycosis pneumonia with erythema nodosum. Close to 70% of all cases of erythema nodosum have an identified cause (infection, drugs, systemic illness, pregnancy). Common causes include streptococcal infection, sarcoidosis, lymphoma, and inflammatory bowel disease. NSAIDs are helpful in treating the inflammation of erythema nodosum. However, once an underlying cause for erythema nodosum has been identified, treatment of that cause, in this case fluconazole for fungal pneumonia, is indicated (**E**).

Erythema Nodosum

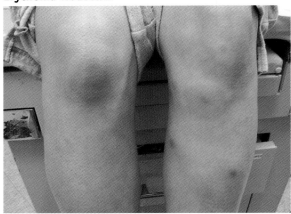

Erythema nodosum is an acute inflammatory, immunologic reaction to the subcutaneous fat characterized by the appearance of painful nodules in the lower legs. It represents a reaction pattern to a variety of etiologic agents, including drugs, infections, and other inflammatory or immunologic diseases. Lesions tend to be bright red, nodular, and tender to palpation, and are often accompanied by fever and malaise.

- Multiple and diverse etiologies: drugs, infections, inflammatory or granulomatous disease
- Painful, tender lesions on lower legs for a few days' duration accompanied by fever, malaise, and arthralgia (commonly ankles)
- Management is symptomatic (bed rest, compression bandages) or directed at the etiology, when identified (antiinflammatory drugs, glucocorticoids).
- Women are affected more than men (10:1 ratio).

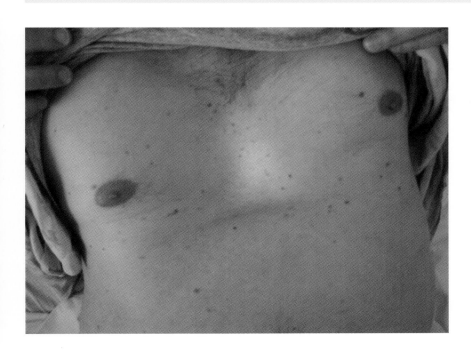

 Notes

63. A 25-year-old man with a history of mitral valve prolapse (MVP) presents with 1 day of sharp, tearing chest pain at the center of his chest that now radiates toward his neck. Physical exam reveals low blood pressure, moderate sternal depression, and a tall, thin man with long arms. What is likely to be abnormal in this patient?

A. Collagen
B. Fibrillin 1
C. LDL cholesterol
D. HDL cholesterol
E. Urine homocystine level

✎ *Notes*

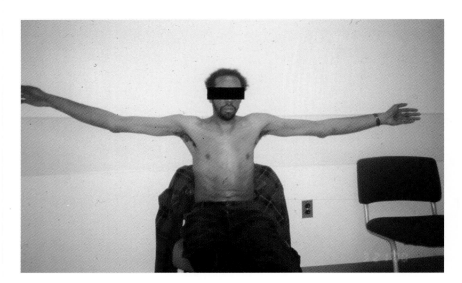

64. A 16-year-old man presents to his primary care physician with a complaint of "near-sightedness." He reports that he has recently had difficulty reading signs and discerning faces at a distance. The patient is a very tall, thin man with long arms and fingers. Physical exam reveals moderate sternal depression and striae distensae on the shoulder and axillary area. On visual acuity exam the patient is found to have 20/100 OD and 20/80 OS vision. What additional screening test will not be necessary in this patient?

A. Annual ophthalmic exam
B. Urine homocystine level
C. Annual echocardiograms
D. Annual chest x-ray
E. Annual musculoskeletal evaluation for kyphoscoliosis

63. **The answer is B: Fibrillin 1.** This patient is having an aortic dissection and has classic findings of Marfan syndrome, including MVP, long arms, and pectus excavatum. Marfan syndrome is caused by a defect in fibrillin 1 (**B**). Collagen defects (**A**) are associated with Ehlers-Danlos syndrome, in which patients exhibit skin hyperextensibility and joint hypermobility. Low LDL and high HDL cholesterol (**C** and **D**) would put a patient at risk for an acute coronary syndrome. Urine homocystine abnormalities (**E**) can be seen in homocystinuria, a recessively inherited metabolic disorder that can lead to ectopia lentis, mental retardation, bone overgrowth, and a high predisposition to thromboembolism and coronary artery disease in the absence of aortic root dilation.

64. **The answer is D: Annual chest x-ray.** This patient exhibits many of the classic features of Marfan syndrome, including myopia, long limbs, arachnodactyly, striae distensae, and pectus excavatum. Marfan syndrome is a generalized disorder of connective tissue caused by a defect in fibrillin 1 that has primary manifestations in the skeletal, ocular, and cardiovascular systems. As a result, Marfan patients commonly suffer from disorders in these systems and must be closely screened. Annual ophthalmic exams (**A**), including slit-lamp examination, are necessary to screen for ectopia lentis, an upward displacement of the lens affecting up to 70% of patients with Marfan syndrome, which may lead to dislocation and acute glaucoma. Urine homocystine levels (**B**) should be checked in all patients suspected of having Marfan syndrome to rule out homocystinuria, a recessively inherited metabolic disorder that can lead to similar clinical manifestations as Marfan syndrome, including ectopia lentis. Annual echocardiograms (**C**) are indicated in all patients with Marfan syndrome to screen for MVP and dilation of the proximal aorta, which can lead to aortic dissection. Annual musculoskeletal evaluation for kyphoscoliosis (**E**) is particularly important in younger patients who are still growing, as severe kyphoscoliosis is frequently seen in Marfan syndrome. An annual chest x-ray (**D**) is not a recommended screening test for patients with Marfan syndrome.

Marfan Syndrome

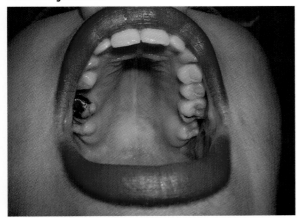

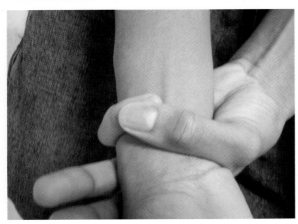

Marfan syndrome is an autosomal dominant disorder of connective tissue protein, fibrillin 1. Abnormal connective tissue development may result in cardiovascular, musculoskeletal, skin, lung, and CNS abnormalities. Musculoskeletal features include: long limbs, arachnodactyly, pectus excavatum or carinatum, scoliosis, high arched palate, high pedal arches, and joint hypermobility. Cardiovascular features include MVP, aortic root dilation, aortic dissection, and rupture. Ocular features include superior lens dislocation and retinal detachment. A diagnosis of Marfan syndrome should also be considered in patients with recurrent spontaneous pneumothoraces secondary to rupture of blebs.

- FBN1 gene
- Fibrillin 1 protein
- Affects about 1 in 5000 people in the United States
- Treat with β-blockers to decrease myocardial contractility and slow rate of aortic dissection
- Routine echocardiogram monitoring to evaluate aortic root diameter

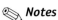 *Notes*

_____

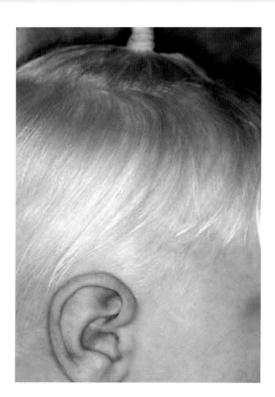

65. A 25-year-old Caucasian mother brings her 4-week-old girl to the office. She expresses concern that her daughter appears different than she and the father. The baby's skin is "snow white," as are her eyebrows and scalp hair. She appears well and exhibits normal development. Her pale blue irides are translucent, and the corneal light reflex is asymmetric. Nystagmus is present. Which advice should be given to the mother regarding her daughter's condition?

A. She is likely to have lower-than-average intelligence and behavioral problems.
B. Obtain a peripheral blood smear.
C. Preventive measures to minimize the risk of sun damage should be initiated when she reaches puberty.
D. She should be under the care of an ophthalmologist and dermatologist in addition to her primary care physician.
E. She should have emergent genetic testing.

66. A 10-month-old Caucasian boy has recurrent skin and lung infections. His skin and hair are white, and his face has a pink hue. His mother says he's the first "albino" in the family. A recent workup revealed neutropenia and neutrophils with large grayish-blue granules. Which of the following is the most appropriate treatment?

A. Regular transfusions
B. Splenectomy
C. Bone marrow transplant
D. IV immunoglobulin
E. Reassurance

65. The answer is D: She should be under the care of an ophthalmologist and dermatologist in addition to her primary care physician. The infant has oculocutaneous albinism (OCA), evident by her white skin and hair, as well as iris translucency, nystagmus, and other ocular abnormalities. People with OCA have an increased risk of skin cancer, most commonly squamous cell carcinoma, and vision problems. Therefore they should be followed by a dermatologist and ophthalmologist (**D**). OCA results from a defect in melanin synthesis, causing obvious skin and hair manifestations, as well as less obvious but pathognomonic translucent irides and nystagmus. Iris translucency is best seen in a dark room with a flashlight shined at the sclera. Preventive measures to decrease sun exposure should be initiated at birth (**C**). OCA is not associated with cognitive or behavioral problems (**A**). Albinism may result from a number of genetic mutations, which can be identified with genetic testing; however, this is unlikely to affect management (**E**). In addition, there are special types of albinism associated with hematologic abnormalities, such as Hermansky-Pudlak syndrome and Chédiak-Higashi syndrome, but the patient in this case does not appear to have one of these syndromes (**B**).

66. The answer is C: Bone marrow transplant. Chédiak-Higashi syndrome is a rare autosomal recessive disorder that presents with oculocutaneous albinism and neutropenia. Giant grayish-blue granules are seen in neutrophils. The preferred treatment is bone marrow transplant (**C**). Patients with Chédiak-Higashi have recurrent pyogenic infections. Common organisms include *S. aureus, S. pyogenes,* and *Pseudomonas*. Patients with Chédiak-Higashi syndrome may have mild bleeding, but regular transfusions are not indicated (**A**). IV immunoglobulin is appropriate for some antibody-related immunodeficiencies (**D**). There is no role for splenectomy in the management of Chédiak-Higashi syndrome (**B**). Chédiak-Higashi syndrome is a serious condition that warrants aggressive management as it often results in death before the age of 7 if untreated (**E**).

Albinism

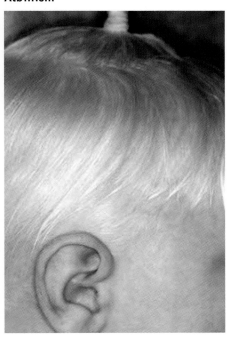

Albinism is most commonly due to autosomal recessive mutations in melanin synthesis. It is present at birth and typically affects the eyes and skin (OCA). In OCA, there is a normal number of melanocytes, but a key enzyme in melanin synthesis, tyrosinase, is inactive.

- Typical features: white skin and hair, including eyelashes and eyebrows; translucent irides and nystagmus are pathognomonic
- Nystagmus is due to foveal hypoplasia with decreased visual acuity and altered optic nerve formation.
- Some fair-skinned people may appear to have albinism, but absence of iris translucency and nystagmus differentiates them from individuals with the disorder.
- Early diagnosis of albinism is essential to minimizing the incidence of skin cancer so that patients can take preventive measures to limit sun exposure.

✎ *Notes*

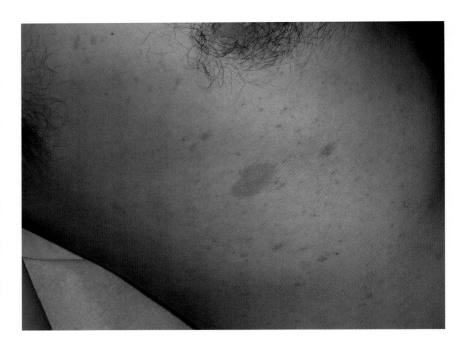

67. A 16-year-old man presents with complaints of a rash. During the physical examination, you note multiple tiny, symmetric papules and plaques, most prominent over the trunk. A single larger lesion is present over the patient's side. This lesion is salmon colored with a central scale located within the oval plaque. What is the best treatment for this rash?

A. No treatment is needed. It should resolve in 6-8 weeks.
B. Topical antifungal treatment
C. Oral antifungal treatment
D. Topical nystatin
E. Topical hydrocortisone cream

68. A 23-year-old woman with no past medical history presents complaining of a 1-week history of an itchy rash on her back and abdomen. She notes that the rash initially began as a single larger patch on her abdomen one week ago. She has not recently started any new medications or changed her detergents or soaps. On physical exam the patient has several erythematous, fine, scaling plaques and patches ranging from 1-3 cm with fine collarette scales at the periphery of each lesion. What is the most likely diagnosis of this patient's rash?

A. Secondary syphilis
B. Guttate psoriasis
C. Erythema multiforme (EM)
D. Pityriasis rosea
E. Tinea corporis

67. **The answer is A: No treatment is needed. It should resolve in 6-8 weeks.** This patient has classic findings of pityriasis rosea, including a herald patch and a rash most prominent over the trunk. Because this is thought to be due to a reaction to human herpesvirus (HHV) infection, the viral exanthem should resolve spontaneously in 6-8 weeks (**A**). Herald patches may be confused with ringworm; however, the scale of a herald patch is classically located inside the patch. In ringworm, which is caused by tinea, the scale is located outside the patch. Ringworm is due to a fungal infection and is most often treated with topical antifungals (**B**). In some cases, such as tinea capitis, an oral antifungal treatment (**C**) may be needed. Topical nystatin (**D**) is often used to treat candida infections. Topical hydrocortisone cream (**E**) is not needed to treat this viral exanthem.

68. **The answer is D: Pityriasis rosea.** This patient presents with the characteristic symptoms of pityriasis rosea (**D**), including an initial herald patch (a 2- to 5-cm, salmon-red patch that is the presenting symptom in 80% of patients) with a scale located inside the patch. This is in contrast to tinea corporis (**E**) that presents with scaling lesions with scales located outside the patch. Secondary syphilis presents as a papulosquamous truncal eruption that involves the palms and soles, which is not seen in this patient. Guttate psoriasis (**B**) is characterized by eruption of small (0.5-1.5 cm) papules over the upper trunk and proximal extremities. These lesions are much smaller than those in pityriasis and do not present with a herald patch. EM (**C**) presents as target lesions that may coalesce and develop erosions over the body in response to herpes simplex virus (HSV) and certain drugs.

Pityriasis Rosea

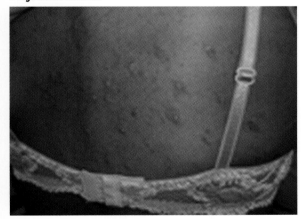

Pityriasis rosea is an acute viral exanthem and manifests with a characteristic skin rash. The rash begins with a herald patch, a single scaly salmon-colored 2- to 5-cm oval lesion. After 1-2 weeks, a secondary eruption of smaller fine scaling papules and plaques with collarettes evolves.

The secondary exanthem is distributed symmetrically in a Christmas tree–like pattern most prominent over the trunk, neck, and adjacent extremities. The long axis of these oval lesions tends to be oriented with the cleavage lines of the skin. Of note, the initial herald patch may be confused with tinea. Pityriasis rosea's scale is located within the oval plaque, whereas tinea's scale is located at the border of the oval plaque. Pityriasis rosea is typically self-limiting and resolves within 6-8 weeks. Treatment is usually not needed, but topical zinc oxide, calamine lotion, or moderate potency corticosteroids can be used for pruritis.

- Herald patch
- Christmas tree–like rash
- Scale located within oval plaque
- Self-limiting
- Thought to be a reaction to HHV 7

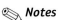

Notes _____

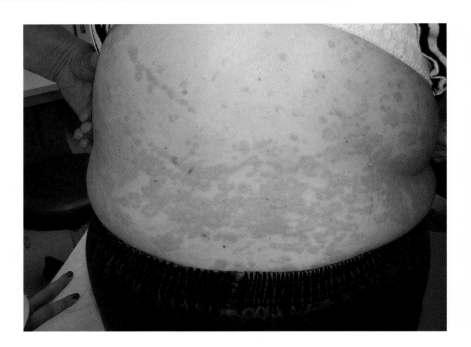

69. A 19-year-old man presents with edematous, pruritic papules on his abdomen and chest. The lesions appeared shortly after eating a shellfish meal at a restaurant. He also complains of difficulty breathing and swallowing and has wheezing on examination. What is the most appropriate treatment for this patient?

A. Benadryl
B. Topical glucocorticoids
C. Systemic glucocorticoids
D. Intramuscular (IM) epinephrine
E. Ranitidine

70. A 23-year-old woman comes to the urgent care center complaining of a rash around her neck. For Valentine's Day, her fiancé gave her a beautiful gold necklace. Since wearing this necklace, she has developed a skin rash notable for pale-red, raised, itchy papules and vesicles around her neck. You suspect that she has developed contact dermatitis from her necklace. Which of the following is the most likely mechanism of her rash development?

A. Type 4 delayed cell-mediated hypersensitivity
B. Immune complex disease
C. Cytotoxic, antibody-dependent response
D. Type 1 hypersensitivity reaction
E. Release of histamine from eosinophils

69. The answer is D: IM epinephrine. This patient is having a severe allergic reaction to shellfish. He has urticaria as well as signs of angioedema and airway constriction. Thus this patient should be given IM epinephrine (**D**). Benadryl (**A**) is an H1 blocker and ranitidine (**E**) is an H2 blocker. Although they are both antihistamines, epinephrine should be used as first line treatment if there are signs of airway compromise. Systemic glucocorticoids (**C**) can be used to alleviate urticaria, but would not be first line in this situation. Topical glucocorticoids (**B**) may help to alleviate the itching associated with urticaria and may help the lesions resolve, but this patient is showing concerning signs of systemic inflammation. This patient should be instructed to avoid shellfish and should carry an EpiPen in the future.

70. The answer is A: Type 4 delayed cell-mediated hypersensitivity. This woman is experiencing an allergic contact dermatitis, a type 4 hypersensitivity reaction (**A**). Her collar-like rash is confined to the area of allergen exposure, in this case nickel sulfate. Immune complex disease (**B**) is a type 3 hypersensitivity reaction, characteristic of an arthus reaction or serum sickness. Cytotoxic, antibody-dependent reactions (**C**) are type 2 hypersensitivity reactions. Examples include autoimmune hemolytic anemia and erythroblastosis fetalis. Type 1 hypersensitivity reaction (**D**) is characteristic of anaphylaxis and asthma. Histamine is not released from eosinophils (**E**).

Urticaria

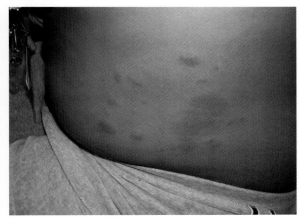

Urticaria, commonly called *hives,* are due to either an allergic and nonallergic stimuli that causes the release of inflammatory mediators, including histamine and mast cells. Urticaria can result from contact dermatitis, food, drugs, recent upper respiratory infections, and environmental factors. Key features include evanescent wheals (raised areas surrounded by a red base) or hives. Itching is usually intense. Most incidences are acute and self-limited. Lesions typically last less than 24 hours. Chronic urticaria is defined as recurrent episodes lasting longer than 6 weeks. Urticaria may be associated with angioedema, flushing, burning, wheezing, and abdominal pain. Antihistamines and prednisone are the mainstays of treatment. If angioedema and wheezing are prominent, IM epinephrine may also be used.

- Histamine and mast cells
- Most common causes: food, drugs, contact dermatitis
- Chronic urticaria >6 weeks

Notes

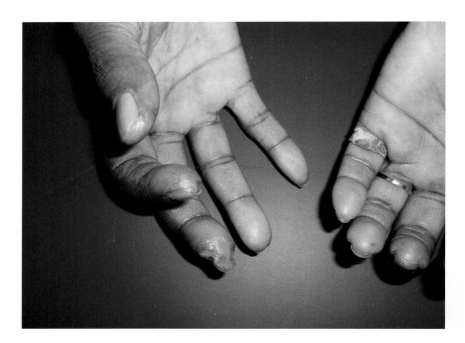

71. A 41-year-old woman presents with painful ulcerations of her distal fingers. On physical examination she also has nail fold capillary changes and tight thickened skin over her hands, causing loss of mobility of her fingers. Which of the following would help to confirm the diagnosis?

A. Anticentromere antibodies
B. Anti–double-stranded DNA (anti-dsDNA) antibodies
C. Anti-Smith (anti-Sm) antibodies
D. Antineutrophil cytoplasmic antibody (ANCA) levels
E. Biopsy of the ulcerations

72. A 52-year-old man presents with a change in his facial appearance. He has noticed tightening of the skin around his mouth and eyebrows. In addition, his fingers have developed a sausage-like appearance. Two years ago he had been diagnosed with Raynaud phenomenon (RP). He recalls his mother suffering from a condition severely affecting the mobility of her fingers. Which of the following is the most accurate regarding this patient's likely diagnosis?

A. Women are four times as likely as men to develop the disease.
B. Positive anti-dsDNA and anti-Sm antibodies confirm the condition.
C. The condition can be cured with agents used to increase blood flow to the affected areas.
D. RP is a result of chronic disease progression.
E. This familial condition can be mapped to the short arm of chromosome 3.

71. **The answer is D: ANCA levels.** This patient has digital ulceration due to vasculitis caused by RP. In this case, the RP is likely secondary to scleroderma given the physical exam findings of nail fold capillary changes and sclerodactyly. ANA (antinuclear antibodies), anti-Scl, and anticentromere antibodies (**A**) are helpful in diagnosing scleroderma. Anticentromere antibody is specific for CREST, a limited form of scleroderma. Anti-dsDNA antibodies (**B**) and anti-Sm (**C**) antibodies are positive in lupus. Lupus patients may also experience RP, but the physical exam findings in this patient are consistent with scleroderma, not lupus. ANCA levels (**D**) can be positive in certain conditions causing vasculitis. Cytoplasmic antineutrophil cytoplasmic antibody (C-ANCA) is positive in conditions such as Wegener syndrome. Perinuclear antineutrophil cytoplasmic antibodies (P-ANCA) may be positive in Churg-Strauss syndrome, primary sclerosing cholangitis, and polyarteritis nodosa. A biopsy (**E**) of the ulceration will show necrosis but would not be helpful in determining a cause.

72. **The answer is A: Women are four times as likely as men to develop the disease.** This patient has scleroderma. Scleroderma is four times as likely in women compared to men (**A**). RP is an early manifestation of disease, and many patients will present with Raynaud (**D**). Positive anti-dsDNA and anti-Sm antibodies suggest lupus (**B**). Scleroderma is a chronic autoimmune condition without a cure. Treatment is aimed at alleviating symptoms (**C**). The cause of scleroderma is unknown, and while symptoms seem to run in families, a specific gene has not yet been identified.

Scleroderma (Hands)

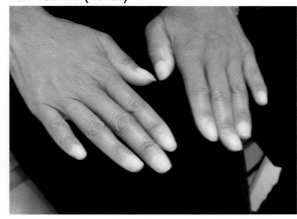

Scleroderma is a chronic autoimmune disease characterized by fibrosis, vascular alterations, and autoantibodies. Limited scleroderma mainly affects the hands, arms, and face. Facial involvement may include a smooth, unwrinkled brow, tight area around the nose, and a shrunken, expressionless mouth. Involved skin feels smooth and indurated and as if it is bound to underlying structures. Areas of hyperpigmentation or hypopigmentation may be present.

CREST syndrome is an example of limited scleroderma, which results in *C*alcinosis, *R*aynaud phenomenon, *E*sophageal dysfunction, *S*clerodactyly (fibrosed skin causes immobile digits), and *T*elangiectasias. Pulmonary arterial hypertension is the most serious complication of this form of scleroderma. Limited scleroderma can also cause vascular changes in the extremities, such as the hands, which may lead to local ulcerations and digit ischemia. Diffuse scleroderma is rapidly progressing and affects large areas of skin and at least one internal organ—frequently the kidneys, esophagus, heart, and lungs. Fibrosis and tightening of the skin may result in flexion contractures.

- Ninety-five percent of cases have positive ANA. Anti-Scl has lower sensitivity, but higher specificity.
- Anticentromere is 80% sensitive for CREST syndrome.
- Treatment: immunosuppressive agents, such as methotrexate
- Hand findings in scleroderma: Raynaud, sclerodactyly, nail fold capillary changes
- RP is seen in approximately 90% of patients.
- Women are affected three to four times more frequently than men.

Notes

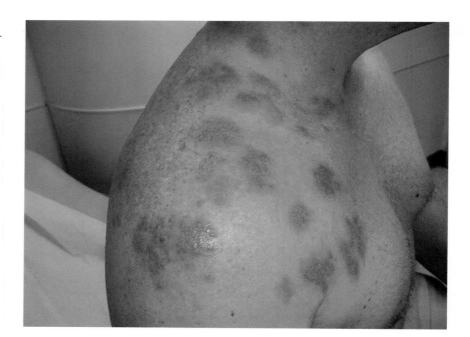

73. A healthy 58-year-old man comes to the clinic because of a rash over his neck and shoulder. He states that he started having a burning pain sensation in the area one day prior to the rash appearing. He has been experiencing many life changes recently, as his company closed and he has been out of work for 1 month. On physical examination, the rash is located on the right aspect of the neck, over the right clavicle and right deltoid area in the C3-C4 dermatomes. What measure(s) can be taken to decrease his risk of postherpetic neuralgia?

A. Early institution of antiinflammatory medications
B. Early antiviral therapy including valacyclovir 1 g bid
C. Administer zoster vaccine now
D. All of the above

74. A 23-year-old female graduate student presents to the office the day after defending her thesis. She complains that 2 days ago she felt a tingling, pulsing, right-sided headache. It gradually turned into an intense burning pain over her right forehead, and then she noticed red bumps over that area. On exam, vesicles of varying size are seen erupting from an erythematous base in the superior dermatome of the right cranial nerve (CN) V_1 with minimal periorbital involvement. The rash extends over the right forehead and scalp to the vertex, overlapping the midline by only 1 cm. This patient is diagnosed clinically with herpes zoster ophthalmicus. Which of the following is/are true regarding this condition?

A. Early antiviral therapy can reduce extent of eruption and sequelae.
B. High risk for corneal involvement, lid involvement, and uveitis
C. Associated with a prodrome of headaches, nausea, and vomiting
D. All of the above

73. **The answer is B: Early antiviral therapy including valacyclovir 1 g bid.** This patient is suffering from herpes zoster in the C3 and C4 dermatomes. This rash represents reactivation of latent varicella-zoster virus from the spinal ganglia. It reaches the skin through sensory nerves and therefore presents in a dermatomal pattern of erythematous maculopapular clusters of vesicles. An important potential consequence is postherpetic neuralgia, which represents chronic pain in the affected nerves due to inflammatory damage during reactivation. Limiting the duration and spread of the reaction are important in the acute phase, and administration of the zoster vaccine to appropriate patients can reduce the incidence of postherpetic neuralgia by two thirds (**E**).

74. **The answer is D: All of the above.** This patient has herpes zoster ophthalmicus along the CN V$_1$ dermatome (right ophthalmic branch of the trigeminal nerve) most likely brought on by stress. She had a prodromal headache. Other aspects of the prodrome include nausea, vomiting, and preauricular/submaxillary lymphadenopathy. Although she is at risk for ocular involvement, this herpes zoster eruption is primarily in the frontal branch of CN V$_1$. The highest risk for serious ocular complications is with eruption along the nasociliary branch of CN V$_1$, which innervates the tip and side of the nose and the eye (Hutchinson sign). Early antiviral therapy (valacyclovir, acyclovir, famciclovir) can decrease eruption, ocular involvement, and postherpetic neuralgia (**D**).

Herpes Zoster

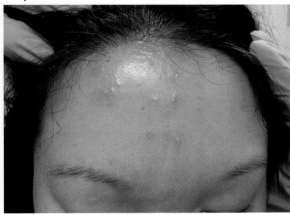

Herpes zoster is caused by the varicella-zoster virus that causes chickenpox. Herpes zoster is classically characterized by unilateral, dermatomal pain and rash as a result of reactivation of the latent varicella-zoster virus in the spinal ganglia. Erythematous, vesicular, maculopapular lesions appear in clusters in a dermatomal distribution. Pain is the most important clinical manifestation, and the patient may experience chronic pain from postherpetic neuralgia after resolution of the rash. A varicella-zoster vaccine reduces the incidence of herpes zoster by one half and the incidence of postherpetic neuralgia by two thirds.

- Latent varicella-zoster virus reactivating and traveling to skin in dermatomal pattern via sensory nerves
- Elderly and immunosuppressed individuals are most commonly affected.
- Antiviral therapy and analgesia are helpful in the acute setting.
- Goals of therapy are limitation of pain and rash duration acutely, limiting disease spread, and preventing postherpetic neuralgia.
- Postherpetic neuralgia treatment can include lidocaine patches, oral gabapentin, and tricyclic antidepressants.

✎ *Notes*

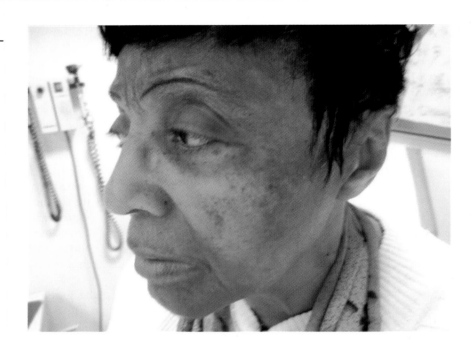

75. A 54-year-old woman with a family history of osteoporosis and a 40–pack year smoking history until 2 years ago was recently started on a combined estrogen and progesterone regimen to prevent osteoporosis. She now returns to the clinic complaining of new-onset dark patches of skin on her face. She notes that she has recently been spending several hours in the sun every day tending her garden. On physical exam, the patient exhibits symmetric macular hyperpigmentation on her cheeks and forehead. What is the most likely diagnosis of this patient's hyperpigmentation?

A. Postinflammatory hypermelanotic macules
B. Systemic lupus erythematosus (SLE)
C. Melasma
D. Vitiligo
E. Hypersensitivity reaction to combined hormone replacement therapy (HRT)

76. A 31-year-old G1P0 woman presents with complaints of dark patches of skin on her face. This is the first time she has experienced these lesions, and she notes that her skin has always been healthy. The lesions have appeared gradually, but they have become more visible in the last month. You note hyperpigmented patches over her cheeks, upper lip, and forehead. What advice would you give this patient?

A. Begin topical therapy with hydrocortisone cream
B. Begin topical therapy with progesterone cream
C. Refer her to dermatologist for a biopsy
D. Recommend that she avoids exposure to sunlight
E. Reassure her that the lesions are benign and are commonly associated with aging

75. **The answer is C: Melasma.** This patient is most likely experiencing melasma (**C**), an acquired light- or dark-brown hyperpigmentation resulting from exposure to sunlight combined with the initiation of HRT. Melasma occurs most commonly in women, and only about 10% of patients are males. The disorder is very common, particularly among pregnant women and women taking combination estrogen and progesterone therapy who are exposed to sunlight. Melasma does not occur in women taking unopposed estrogen therapy. Postinflammatory hypermelanotic macules (**A**) may resemble this patient's disorder but occur in patients following an inflammatory response such as a drug eruption, psoriasis, or lichen planus. SLE (**B**) may also present with the characteristic malar rash on women in this patient's age group. However, this diagnosis is much less likely given the absence of any family or personal history of SLE and the recent initiation of HRT. Vitiligo (**D**) presents in a distribution similar to melasma. However, the presentation is that of a complete absence of melanocytes and resulting hyp*o*pigmentation as opposed to the hyp*er*pigmentation seen in melasma. This patient's presentation could be seen following a drug eruption (**E**) as postinflammatory hypermelanotic macules but would not be the initial presentation of a hypersensitivity reaction.

76. **The answer is D: Recommend that she avoids exposure to sunlight.** This patient has melasma, also called *the mask of pregnancy* when it occurs in pregnant patients. Sunlight accentuates the hyperpigmentation, and patients should be advised to avoid sun exposure as much as possible (**D**). Topical therapy with hydroquinone cream can be used to lighten areas of hyperpigmentation, but topical therapy with hydrocortisone cream (**A**) would not be beneficial. Hormones during pregnancy, such as estrogen and progesterone, are thought to stimulate melanocytes, thus a topical progesterone cream (**B**) would not be helpful. There is no need for biopsy (**C**) as the lesions are benign and typically fade once pregnancy has ended or hormonal therapy is stopped. These lesions are not commonly associated with aging (**E**). They are associated with pregnancy, combined HRT, and hormonal contraception that contains both estrogen and progesterone.

Melasma

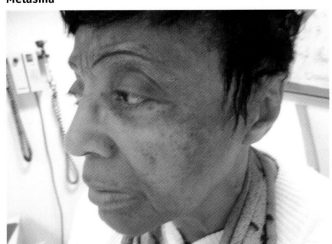

Melasma, also known as *the mask of pregnancy* when present in pregnant women, is a tan or dark skin discoloration. The dark patches are commonly seen on the cheeks, nose, upper lip, and forehead areas. Melasma is more common in women, especially pregnant women and those taking combined oral or patch contraceptives or HRT. The combination of estrogen and progesterone are thought to stimulate melanocytes. Sunlight accentuates this hyperpigmentation. The lesions typically fade after stopping hormone therapy or at the cessation of pregnancy.

- Masklike hyperpigmentation on face
- More often seen in women during pregnancy or in women taking combined estrogen and progesterone
- Sunlight accentuates pigmentation
- Treatment: minimize sun exposure or apply hydroquinone cream (works for any hyperpigmentation)

Notes

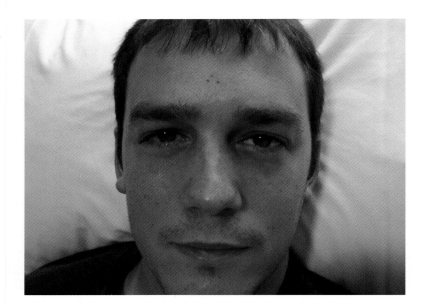

77. A 24-year-old man comes to the clinic for an eruption on his face, back, neck, and the dorsa of his hands. In the past he was told the rash on his face was seborrhea and was treated with topical glucocorticoids. He also complains of 2 months of fatigue and weakness. He is a graduate student and has difficulty climbing the three flights of stairs to his lecture hall and office. Physical examination reveals a violaceous periorbital rash most prominent on the upper eyelids, erythematous plaques on the posterior shoulders and neck, violaceous papules on the knuckles, and dystrophic nails with telangiectasias present. Muscle strength is 4/5 in all extremities. Which of the following statements regarding this patient is/are true?

A. Diagnosis must be confirmed with testing for antinuclear and myositis-specific antibodies.

B. Shortness of breath is always related to interstitial lung disease.

C. Hallmark skin lesions of heliotrope periorbital rash and Gottren papules are pathognomonic for this disease.

D. Systemic treatment should only be instituted for advanced cases.

E. A and C only

78. A 37-year-old man presents to the clinic with 3 months of difficulty standing once seated and weakness in reaching above his head. He reports some muscle aches and morning joint pain and stiffness. He also complains of difficulty swallowing and shortness of breath with exercise. For the last few weeks the patient has noticed a red rash around his eyes and on his chest and shoulders after a week's vacation at the beach. Physical exam shows a periorbital heliotrope rash, patches of erythema on the posterior shoulders and chest, violaceous papules on the knuckles, and periungual erythema with telangiectasias. Muscle strength is 4/5 in all extremities. Which of the following is/are treatment option(s) for this patient?

A. Decrease sun exposure

B. Hydroxychloroquine

C. Oral prednisone

D. Methotrexate

E. Physical therapy

F. All of the above

77. The answer is C: Hallmark skin lesions of **heliotrope periorbital rash and Gottren papules are pathognomonic for this disease.** This patient has the hallmark signs of dermatomyositis (DM), which include the heliotrope periorbital rash, Gottren papules (violaceous papules on the knuckles), and proximal muscle weakness (**C**). Macular erythema on the posterior shoulders and neck (shawl sign) is also present. Autoantibody testing is not required for the diagnosis but may be of prognostic value. Shortness of breath in a patient with DM can have a variety of causes, including weakness of the muscles of respiration, pulmonary disease (restrictive lung disease, interstitial pneumonitis, aspiration pneumonia, opportunistic infections), and myocardial disease (conduction defects, cardiomyopathy). Early systemic treatment slows the progression of disease and is associated with improved outcomes.

78. The answer is F: All of the above. This patient exhibits cutaneous disease and systemic effects of DM with proximal muscle weakness and esophageal, pulmonary, and joint involvement. Oral prednisone is central to treatment. However, for 25% of patients who will not respond to steroids, adjuvant therapy with methotrexate and other chemotherapy agents (mycophenolate mofetil [MMF], azathioprine, cyclophosphamide) can be used. Patients need physical therapy to prevent muscle atrophy from DM. Cutaneous disease is photosensitive, so both decreasing sun exposure and using sunscreen are key. Additionally, antimalarial medications (hydroxychloroquine) are effective in treating cutaneous DM (**F**).

Dermatomyositis

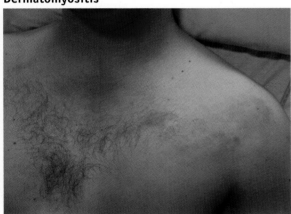

Dermatomyositis (DM) is an autoimmune myopathy that results in skeletal muscle weakness and cutaneous inflammatory disease. It is characterized by violaceous (heliotrope) inflammatory changes of the eyelids and periorbital area, macular erythema of the posterior shoulders and neck (shawl sign), and violaceous or lacy pink Gottren papules over the knuckles. It may have associated polymyositis, interstitial pneumonitis, myocardial disease, and joint disease. Juvenile onset of disease may be associated with vasculitis and calcinosis, while adult-onset (age >55) disease may be related to malignancy. Laboratory tests will show increased serum creatine kinase with muscle disease, and ANA- and myositis-specific autoantibodies may be detected. Treatment is aimed at decreasing exposure to sunlight, local therapy with topical corticosteroids to decrease cutaneous inflammation and pruritus, and systemic therapy consisting of systemic glucocorticoids, hydroxychloroquine, and antihistamines.

- Classic violaceous (heliotrope) rash of periorbital area and eyelids; photosensitivity
- Shawl sign: macular erythema on shoulders, neck, and chest
- Gottren papules are distinct violaceous papules over the DIP joints.
- Progressive proximal muscle weakness manifested by difficulty rising from seated position, raising the arms above the head, and climbing stairs

✎ *Notes*

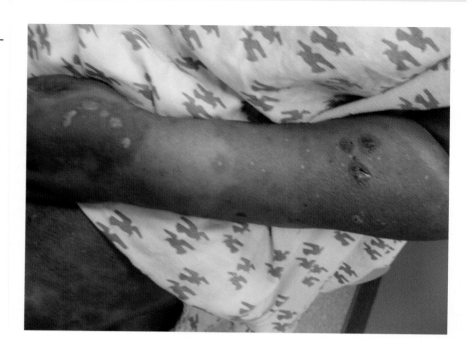

79. A 74-year-old woman presents to your office complaining of blisters on her arms, legs, and lower abdomen. She initially had itching and hives in the area prior to developing the blisters. Her past medical history is remarkable for a urinary tract infection treated with trimethoprim/sulfamethoxazole 1 year ago and prehypertension treated with lifestyle changes. Physical exam reveals tense blisters on the upper arms, forearms, thighs, lower legs, and lower abdomen. No oral lesions are present. Some excoriations are present, and several blisters have ruptured, leaving behind erosions. A biopsy of the lesion reveals a subepidermal blister and superficial dermal infiltrate. Immunostaining of the biopsy shows a linear pattern along the basement membrane. What are the most likely diagnosis and first-line treatment for this patient?

A. Idiopathic bullous pemphigoid; topical corticosteroids and anesthetics
B. Idiopathic bullous pemphigoid; oral glucocorticoids
C. Drug-induced pemphigoid; oral glucocorticoids and discontinuation of offending agent
D. Drug-induced pemphigoid; immunosuppressant therapy only
E. Pemphigus vulgaris (PV); oral glucocorticoids and an immunosuppressant

80. A 63-year-old woman was treated in the office 1 week ago for a urinary tract infection with ciprofloxacin. She now presents with 1-to 2-cm blisters on her abdomen, in her groin, and on the flexor surfaces of her legs. Physical exam shows that, after digital compression, the blisters do not change size, and they do not break. Digital compression of the bony surfaces of the legs does not produce any lesions. What is the most likely diagnosis in this patient?

A. PV
B. Bullous pemphigoid
C. Dermatitis herpetiformis
D. Steven-Johnson syndrome
E. Scalded skin syndrome

79. The answer is B: Idiopathic bullous pemphigoid; oral glucocorticoids. This patient is suffering from idiopathic bullous pemphigoid, which can be self-limiting but may persist for months to years, with exacerbations and remissions. The biopsy shows the classic findings of a subepidermal blister with a superficial dermal infiltrate, and immunofluorescence reveals the characteristic linear pattern that results from autoantibodies against hemidesmosomes that connect basal cells to the basement membrane. Generalized lesions, as in this patient, require oral glucocorticoids (**B**) and/or immunosuppressive agents (azathioprine, MMF, or cyclophosphamide). Localized disease can be treated with topical corticosteroids alone (**A**). Pemphigoid can also be a reaction to a medication, such as sulfa drugs, certain antibiotics, or β-blockers. However, her history sulfa drug use is remote and therefore unlikely to be the cause of her condition (**C, D**).

80. The answer is B: Bullous pemphigoid. This patient is suffering from drug-induced bullous pemphigoid (**B**), which can easily be differentiated from PV (**A**) since the latter is characterized by flaccid, rather than tense, lesions. The flaccid lesions of PV get bigger after digital compression and can be produced by digital compression on boney surfaces (Nikolsky sign). Bullous pemphigoid is characterized by tense lesions, mostly located on flexor surfaces. It is caused by autoantibodies against basement membrane hemidesmosomal glycoproteins and may be either spontaneous or drug-induced. Dermatitis herpetiformis (**C**), which is related to IgA production, is associated with celiac sprue and produces vesicles/blisters that are closely clustered (as in the herpetic lesions, hence the name). Steven-Johnson syndrome (**D**), also referred to as *mucocutaneous syndrome,* is a drug-induced syndrome that produces both cutaneous and mucosal blisters. Blisters are also present in scalded skin syndrome (**E**), which is related to the superantigen toxin produced by *S. aureus*. However, this is unlikely to explain the patient's symptoms in this case, because *S. aureus* is unlikely to be the cause of the patient's urinary tract infection.

Bullous Pemphigoid

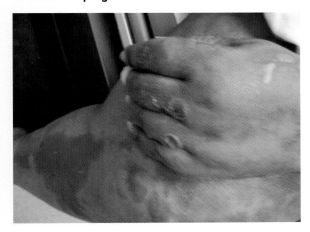

Bullous pemphigoid is an autoimmune disease that causes superficial blistering, usually in patients over age 60. The lesions, which mature from pruritic urticaria to tense bullae, are typically found on the lower abdomen, groin, and flexor surfaces of the extremities, but may be located on the oral mucosa in a minority of patients. As the lesions evolve, the blisters often rupture and are replaced by erosions.

- Histology showing subepidermal blister without epidermal necrosis and a superficial dermal infiltrate containing lymphocytes, histiocytes, and eosinophils
- Immunopathology reveals immunoreactants deposited in a linear pattern along the basement membrane; C3 detected in almost all patients; IgG in most patients as well
- Autoantibodies directed against bullous pemphigoid antigen in the hemidesmosome, which anchors the basal cell to the basement membrane

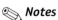

Notes

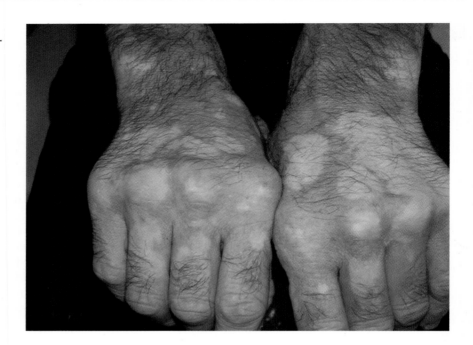

81. A 65-year-old man presents with a 2-week history of white patches of skin on his bilateral hands. They are asymptomatic, and he denies any history of topical medication use. Which of the following is most likely associated with this patient's condition?

A. Guttate hypomelanosis
B. Tinea corporis
C. Pernicious anemia
D. Pityriasis rosea
E. Tinea versicolor

82. A 24-year-old man presents to your office for a routine checkup. He is concerned about the appearance of his skin and requests an explanation for the depigmented areas on his hands and arms. He has had these lesions since birth but notices that they change in shape. What is the most likely explanation for these areas of depigmentation?

A. Overproduction of melanin due to a defect in the TYR gene
B. Destruction or loss of melanocytes of unknown etiology
C. Infection with *Malassezia globosa*
D. Corticosteroid use in infancy
E. Drug reaction to benzoyl peroxide treatment.

81. **The answer is C: Pernicious anemia.** This patient has vitiligo, an acquired loss of pigmentation described histologically by the loss of melanocytes in the epidermis. Vitiligo has been associated with a number of diseases, including pernicious anemia (**C**), stemming from B$_{12}$ deficiency. Guttate hypomelanosis is a benign acquired leukoderma of unknown etiology most commonly seen in middle-aged, light-skinned women (**A**). Fungal infections (**B, D, E**) may have similar appearance to vitiligo, but the patient's associated symptoms make this diagnosis less likely.

82. **The answer is B: Destruction or loss of melanocytes of unknown etiology.** The patient in the vignette most likely has vitiligo, which is due to loss of melanocytes. While the origin of vitiligo is unknown, it may arise from autoimmune, genetic, oxidative stress, neural, or viral causes (**B**). Overproduction of melanocytes would not lead to areas of depigmentation (**A**). Infection with *Malassezia globosa* (**C**) is responsible for the majority of cases of tinea versicolor. Corticosteroid use or benzoyl peroxide treatment (**D, E**) are unlikely to lead to the pictured pattern of hypopigmentation.

Vitiligo

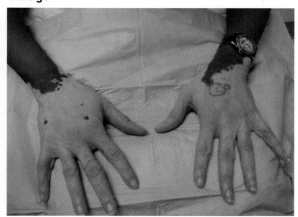

Vitiligo is an acquired loss of pigmentation described histologically by the loss of epidermal melanocytes.

- Associated with autoimmune diseases such as Hashimoto thyroiditis, Addison disease, type 1 diabetes, and pernicious anemia
- The disease is thought to have a hereditary component.
- Commonly involved sites include the face, body folds, and the back of the hands.

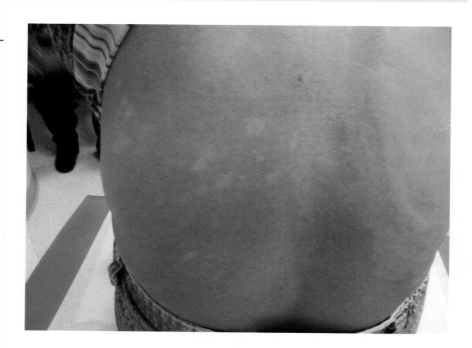

83. A 45-year-old Cambodian woman presents to the refugee clinic with no complaints. On exam, a few discrete large and small hypopigmented macules are noted on the left side of her back. Biopsy reveals large numbers of lymphocytes, low numbers of AFB, and noncaseating granulomas involving nerves. What is the next best step in management of this patient?

A. Oral prednisone
B. Dapsone, clofazimine, and rifampin
C. Sunscreen
D. Gabapentin
E. NSAID

84. A 50-year-old man from India presents to the clinic for routine vaccinations. His past medical history is significant for lepromatous leprosy that was treated 3 years ago. On physical exam, you notice the following: leonine facies; a thickened, palpable left ulnar nerve; a paralyzed, left claw hand with shortened digits; and hypopigmented to erythematous, annular, raised, hypoesthetic plaques throughout his body. Which of the following is/are true regarding lepromatous leprosy?

A. Common sequelae are due to skin infiltration and nerve damage.
B. Causal organism, *Mycobacterium leprae,* is unable to be cultured in vitro.
C. Diagnosed with skin slit smears or skin biopsies
D. Treatment is dapsone, rifampin, and clofazimine for 2 years.
E. All of the above

83. **The answer is B: Dapsone, clofazimine, and rifampin.** This patient has multibacillary, tuberculoid leprosy (TL) with six or more discrete, hypopigmented macules on the left side of her left back. Sensory loss in these lesions is common in TL. *M. leprae* damages peripheral nerves by invading Schwann cells and causing demyelination. Higher numbers of inflammatory lymphocytes (T_H1, CD4+, T cells) in TL limit and control infection but add to nerve damage. The treatment regimen for multibacillary leprosy is dapsone, clofazimine, and rifampin for 2 years (**B**). Side effects include hemolysis with dapsone, orange discoloration of bodily fluids with rifampin, and red to blue skin discoloration with clofazimine.

84. **The answer is E: All of the above.** This patient has burned out, treated lepromatous leprosy (LL), with multiple hypopigmented and erythematous macules, papules and/or nodules with loss of sensation. The disease is caused by *M. leprae,* which is nonamenable to culture to date and endemic primarily in Brazil, India, and parts of Southeast Asia. A classic symptom of LL is leonine facies, thickened skin, and marked skin folds on the face due to dermal infiltration. Nerve damage initiated by Schwann cell invasion causes both cutaneous lesional hypoesthesia and asymmetric peripheral neuropathy (in this case ulnar nerve damage and claw hand). Affected peripheral nerves (ulnar, median, posterior tibial) become inflamed and palpable. Bone infection has caused reabsorption of this patient's left hand digital bones. In the diagnosis of LL, skin slit smears and biopsy would identify many AFB. The treatment regimen for LL is a 2-year course of combined dapsone, rifampin, and clofazimine (**E**). In paucibacillary leprosy, dapsone and rifampin are used for 1 year.

Leprosy

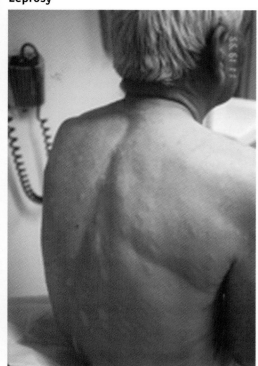

Leprosy (Hansen disease) is a rarely fatal (deaths from amyloidosis and chronic renal failure have been reported), chronic infectious disease caused by *M. leprae*. Clinical manifestations are largely confined to the skin, peripheral nervous system, upper respiratory tract, eyes, and testes. Morbidity is related to this unique tropism and causes characteristic deformities if left untreated. The spectrum of disease from polar tuberculoid to full-blown polar lepromatous disease correlates with symmetric generalized skin manifestations, increasing bacterial load, and loss of T cell–mediated immunity against *M. leprae*. Treatment is with an established regimen of dapsone, clofazimine, and rifampin.

- Leprosy is a disease of the developing world, affecting areas of Asia, Africa, Latin America, and the Pacific.
- TL: least severe form of disease; characterized by a few discrete hypopigmented macules or plaques with absent or low numbers of AFB; asymmetric enlargement of one or a few peripheral nerves may be present
- LL: symmetrically distributed skin nodules, raised plaques, and diffuse dermal infiltration; leonine facies results if the face is involved; AFB are numerous in the skin as well as the peripheral nerves, where they damage both Schwann cells and axons

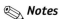 *Notes*

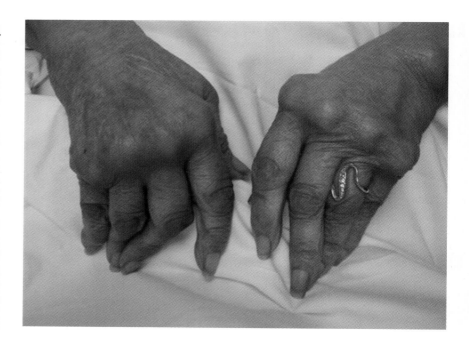

85. A 43-year-old woman presents to your office complaining of a painless nodule on her elbow. This nodule appeared 4 days ago, and the patient cannot recall any trauma or abnormal activity. She denies other symptoms, but as you continue to take a history, the patient recalls pain and crepitus in her wrists for the past 3 years that is relieved with NSAIDs. She usually experiences pain and stiffness in the morning but finds that it is relieved as she goes about her daily activities. The patient is very concerned for malignancy, and you decide to perform a biopsy of the nodule. Which of the following histological patterns is most consistent with rheumatoid arthritis (RA)?

A. Septal panniculitis with acute and chronic inflammation in the fat and around blood vessels

B. A shell of fibrous tissue surrounding a center of fibrinous necrosis

C. Homogeneous eosinophilic staining with hematoxylin and eosin

D. Nodular lesions in the upper dermis composed of calcium phosphate

E. Tumor cells with an elongated shape, intracellular hyaline globs, and high vascularity

86. A 60-year-old woman presents with increasing morning stiffness and pain in her fingers and hands. She has severe tenderness over her metacarpophalangeal (MCP) and proximal interphalangeal (PIP) joints and has had difficulty using her hands due to the pain. She has severe swan neck deformities and boutonniere deformities of her hands. The woman also notes that she has had difficulty breathing and has pain when she takes deep breaths. Which of the following is a risk factor for this disease?

A. HLA-B27 positive

B. HLA-DR4 positive

C. Anti-dsDNA antibodies

D. Anticentromere antibodies

E. Anti-Sm antibodies

85. The correct answer is B: **A shell of fibrous tissue surrounding a center of fibrinous necrosis.** Five percent of patients with RA experience rheumatoid nodules within the first 5 years of diagnosis, and the absolute prevalence of rheumatoid nodules in patients with RA is 25%. Nodules range in size (from pea-sized to the size of a clementine) and are usually subcutaneous, primarily occurring over bony prominences like the knuckles or elbows. Most are painless and cause little to no disability. Histological examination shows a fibrous shell with a center of fibrous necrosis. Smaller nodules tend to be unilocular, while larger nodules are often multilocular, separated by a fibrinous band and containing synovial fluid. Septal panniculitis with acute and chronic inflammation in the fat and around blood vessels (**A**) is consistent with erythema nodosum. Nodules usually occur on the shins and are associated with Homogeneous eosinophilic staining with hematoxylin and eosin (**C**) is consistent with amyloidosis. Nodular lesions in the upper dermis composed of calcium phosphate (**D**) occur in calcinosis cutis, a process of dystrophic calcification that is usually found at sites of previous inflammation or damage to the skin. Tumor cells with an elongated shape, high vascularity, and intracellular hyaline globs are consistent with Kaposi sarcoma.

86. The correct answer is B: **HLA-DR4 positive.** This woman has RA. She has classic joint findings and deformities due to the destructive inflammatory arthritis. She is also experiencing pain with deep breathing, which may indicate pleuritis. Pleuritis can be associated with autoimmune diseases such as RA and SLE. HLA-DR4 positive (**B**) patients are at increased risk of RA. Patients who are HLA-B27 positive (**A**) are at increased risk of ankylosing spondylitis. Anti-dsDNA antibodies (**C**) and anti-Sm antibodies (**E**) are highly specific for lupus. Anticentromere antibodies are specific for CREST syndrome.

Rheumatoid Arthritis (RA)

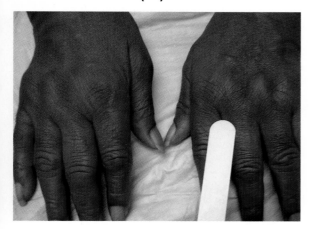

Rheumatoid arthritis (RA) is a chronic systemic inflammatory disorder involving many tissues and organs, particularly the synovial joints. The inflammatory response causes the synovium of the joint to become inflamed and eventually erodes cartilage and bone. In the hands, rheumatoid arthritis may cause joint problems and hand deformities including rheumatoid nodules, swelling, joint stiffness, contractures, ulnar drift, or wrist subluxation. This patient is demonstrating many of the more classic signs of RA in the hand. Boutonniere deformity is hyperextension of the DIP joint and flexion of the PIP joint. Swan neck deformity is flexion of the DIP joint and extension of the PIP joint. RA can also affect larger joints, such as the knees and shoulders. Other findings include rheumatoid nodules, crepitus during movement, and joint swelling. RA can also produce diffuse inflammation in the lungs, pericardium, pleura, and sclera. Onset is most frequent between the ages of 40 and 50, and the disease affects women more than men. X-rays can show narrowing of the joint space, swelling and diminished bone density near the joints, and erosions of the bone. Joint aspiration and blood tests for rheumatoid factor are useful tools to help make the diagnosis. Serologic elevation of rheumatoid factor is often found in RA, but is nonspecific as it is also found in 5% of healthy adults and is associated with a number of other conditions. Treatment for RA is mainly supportive, with the main goals of treatment to relieve pain and restore function to the joints. NSAIDs and oral steroids can help decrease inflammation, relieve pain, and slow progression of the disease. Several disease-modifying treatments are now available, including antimalarial drugs, methotrexate, cyclosporine, gold, remicade, and enbrel. Physical therapy, splints, and warm wax (paraffin) baths may provide some relief.

- Rheumatoid nodules consist of a shell of fibrous tissue surrounding a center of fibrinoid necrosis.
- Swan neck deformities and boutonniere deformities are classic deformities of the hands in patients with RA.
- Findings include chronic synovitis with pannus formation and hyperplasia of synovial cells.
- Morning stiffness, joint pain that is worse after a period of rest and is often relieved with activity
- Usually symmetric and most commonly affects hands and feet
- Higher risk of RA if HLA-DR4 positive

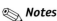 *Notes*

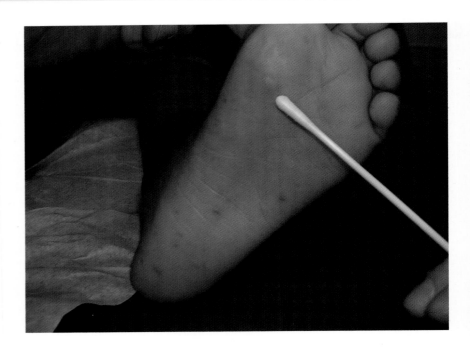

87. A 7-year-old girl is brought to the clinic by her mother, who states she has a fever and has refused to eat over the past 2 days. The patient admits she does not feel well, and her mouth hurts when she eats food. Physical examination reveals a temperature of 100.4° F (38° C); oral vesicles and ulcerations with surrounding erythema on the tongue, gingiva, and buccal mucosa; and gray vesicles on her palms and soles (shown above). Which of the following is the most likely cause of the patient's symptoms?

A. Coxsackievirus group A
B. Poliovirus
C. HSV
D. Rickettsial organism
E. Echovirus

88. A toddler is brought to the clinic by his father who is concerned about spots that suddenly appeared on his son's hands and feet. The toddler recently started going to a daycare center. The father notes that his son hasn't been eating as much as usual the past 2 days. The toddler has a temperature of 100.7° F (38.2° C). There are vesicles on his hands and feet, as well as in his mouth. Which of the following is true of the toddler's condition?

A. He is likely to have febrile seizures.
B. He is likely to develop sepsis.
C. He is likely to develop encephalopathy.
D. He is likely to develop thrombocytopenia.
E. He is unlikely to develop complications, as the disease is typically self-limited.

87. **The answer is A: Coxsackievirus group A.** This patient has hand-foot-and-mouth disease caused by coxsackievirus group A, a single-stranded RNA enterovirus (**A**). This disease is transmitted by the fecal-oral route and is characterized by a prodrome of fever, anorexia, and malaise, followed 1-2 days later by the characteristic lesions in the mouth and on the hands and feet. The initial lesions appear in the mouth as 4- to 8-mm vesicles with an erythematous base, which later ulcerate. They are located on the tongue, soft palate, gingiva, and buccal mucosa. Lesions on the palms and soles appear shortly afterward as red papules that progress to gray vesicles. Treatment is supportive, and the lesions heal in 7-10 days.

88. **The answer is E: He is unlikely to develop complications, as the disease is typically self-limited.** The toddler has hand-foot-and-mouth disease, which is a self-limited condition caused by coxsackievirus group A. Sudden eruption of vesicles on the palms and soles and in the mouth is pathognomonic for hand-foot-and-mouth disease. He is unlikely to develop serious complications (**A, B, C, D**) and will recover on his own in approximately 10 days (**E**).

Coxsackievirus

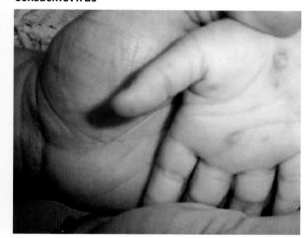

Coxsackievirus is an important cause of illness in young children. It is an enterovirus spread through the oral-oral and fecal-oral routes that causes hand-foot-and-mouth disease. The rash characteristically presents on the palms and soles, as well as in the mouth, as rhomboid or square vesicular lesions with erythematous bases.

- Transmission via fecal-oral route
- Group A viruses: hand-foot-and-mouth disease, herpangina, acute hemorrhagic conjunctivitis
- Group B viruses: pleurodynia, myocarditis, pericarditis
- All coxsackieviruses can cause nonspecific upper respiratory infection, febrile rashes, aseptic meningitis, and paralysis, which is often incomplete and reversible.

✎ *Notes*

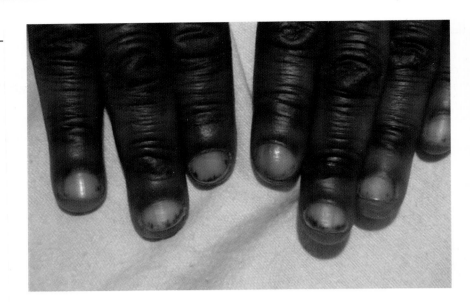

89. A 42-year-old man presents with tiny vertical lines that run under the distal area of his fingernails. They are most prominent on his second and third digits bilaterally. All of the following should be considered in your differential diagnosis except:

A. Microemboli from cholesterol plaque
B. Subacute bacterial endocarditis
C. Subungual melanoma
D. Scleroderma
E. Trauma

90. A 55-year-old man with a history of IV drug use presents to your office complaining of a subjective fever, weakness, and fatigue for the past month. Upon physical exam, you notice small, dark, vertical lines along his nail bed (shown above). Two separate blood cultures are positive for community acquired *S. aureus* in absence of a primary focus. Which of the following criteria would help to fulfill a diagnosis of infective endocarditis?

A. Evidence of endocardial involvement with an echocardiogram demonstrating an intracardiac mass on the tricuspid valve
B. Worsening or changing of a preexisting murmur on physical exam
C. Evidence of conjunctival hemorrhages
D. Nontender, erythematous lesions on the palms and soles
E. Temperature over 37.5° C

89. The answer is C: Subungual melanoma. All of the following are part of the differential diagnosis for splinter hemorrhages, which are tiny lines that run vertically under the distal nails, except subungual melanoma (**C**). Although subungual melanomas are dark vertical lines along the nail, it is rare to have multiple digits involved, and the lesions would not be more likely to occur in the distal nail. Microemboli (**A**), subacute bacterial endocarditis (**B**), and trauma (**E**) may all cause splinter hemorrhages. In addition, systemic vasculitis due to scleroderma (**D**), SLE, or RA can also cause splinter hemorrhages, which result from rupture of nailbed capillaries.

90. The answer is A: Evidence of endocardial involvement with an echocardiogram demonstrating an intracardiac mass on the tricuspid valve. The Duke criteria are a collection of major and minor criteria used to establish the diagnosis of endocarditis. There are three ways to reach a diagnosis: two major criteria, one major and three minor criteria, or five minor criteria.

Major criteria include:
- Positive blood culture with a typical microorganism such as *S. aureus* from two separate blood cultures
- Evidence of endocardial involvement via a positive echocardiogram demonstrating an absence, new partial dehiscence of a prosthetic valve, new valvular regurgitation (increase or change in preexisting murmur not sufficient), or intracardiac mass on a valve or supporting structure
- Minor criteria include:
- Predisposing heart condition or evidence of injection drug use
- Fever over 100.4° F (38° C)
- Evidence of vascular embolisation such as Janeway lesions, major arterial emboli, septic pulmonary infarcts, or mycotic aneurysm
- Immunologic phenomena: glomerulonephritis, Osler nodes, Roth spots, rheumatoid factor
- Evidence of active infection with organism consistent with infective endocarditis or positive blood culture not meeting major criteria

This patient has one major criterion and needs another major criterion (**A**) or three additional minor criteria. Evidence of a worsening murmur (**B**) is insufficient to make the diagnosis of endocarditis. **C**, **D**, and **E** all represent minor criteria in insufficient quantity to make the diagnosis.

Splinter Hemorrhage

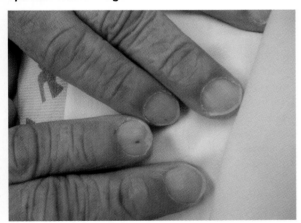

Splinter hemorrhages are tiny lines that run vertically under nails. They are more commonly located in the distal nail plate and represent rupture of nail bed capillaries. This finding is nonspecific, but may due to trauma, a clot from heart (most often due to subacute bacterial endocarditis), cholesterol microemboli, or systemic vasculitis (due to SLE, scleroderma, RA, etc).

- Vertical lines located at distal nail plate
- Due to rupture of nail bed capillaries
- Associated with systemic illnesses, autoimmune diseases, trauma, etc.

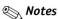
Notes

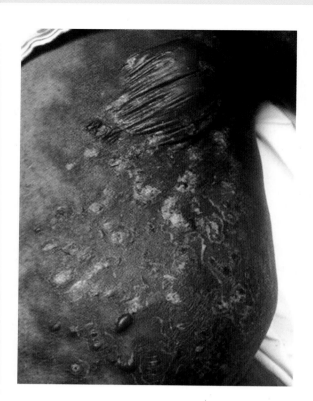

91. A 45-year-old woman presents with painful denuded areas of skin. You note several flaccid bullae that easily rupture when touched. The woman has cutaneous and mucosal lesions. There is a positive Nikolsky sign. What would help to make the diagnosis in this case?

A. Skin biopsy showing immunofluorescence as a linear band along the basement membrane with increased eosinophils in the dermis
B. Skin biopsy showing immunofluorescence surrounding epidermal cells showing tombstone fluorescent pattern
C. Clinical history of herpes infection
D. Wood lamp of urine showing urine fluoresces with distinctive orange-pink color because of increased level of uroporphyrins
E. Recent use of sulfonamides

92. A 48-year-old woman with a history of diet-controlled type 2 diabetes mellitus and hypertension recently started on captopril presents to the ED due to an eruption of painful blisters that began in her mouth and are now present on her torso and back. On physical exam the patient has several painful flaccid bullae on the skin of the torso, and the epidermis is noted to separate with manual pressure applied to these areas. A biopsy of the patient's skin is taken to better discern the diagnosis. Which is the most likely finding on skin biopsy?

A. Subepidermal blisters rich with eosinophils
B. Acantholytic intraepidermal blisters
C. Neutrophil-rich infiltrates within dermal papillae
D. Hydropic degeneration of basal keratinocytes
E. Eosinophilic necrosis of the epidermis

91. **The answer is B: Skin biopsy showing immunofluorescence surrounding epidermal cells showing tombstone fluorescent pattern.** This patient has classic findings of *Pemphigus vulgaris* (PV), including flaccid bullae and positive Nikolsky sign (separation of the epidermis by manual pressure applied to the skin). PV is diagnosed via skin biopsy showing immunofluorescence surrounding epidermal cells leading to a tombstone fluorescent pattern (**B**). A skin biopsy showing immunofluorescence as a linear band along the basement membrane with increased eosinophils in the dermis (**A**) is indicative of bullous pemphigoid. Bullous pemphigoid is an autoimmune process, but presents as hard, tense bullae and a negative Nikolsky sign. A clinical history of herpes infection (**C**) in the setting of blistering may indicate a severe form of EM leading to SJS. EM may be seen following a herpes infection and usually presents with diffuse erythematous target lesions. SJS is a more severe presentation of EM and typically affects mucosal surfaces. Wood lamp of the urine (**D**) would be helpful in diagnosing porphyria cutanea tarda. This condition is due to an autosomal dominant defect in heme synthesis. It can cause blistering, but the blistering is generally confined to sun-exposed areas. Recent use of sulfonamides (**E**) could produce a drug reaction and result in toxic epidermal necrolysis (TEN), which would lead to the widespread loss of sheets of skin. The damage in TEN would involve the entire epidermis.

92. **The answer is B: Acantholytic intraepidermal blisters.** This patient presents with a case of PV, an autoantibody-mediated intraepidermal blistering disease characterized by loss of cohesion between epidermal cells, termed *acantholysis* (**B**). The stimulus for the circulating autoantibodies is often unknown, but PV has been described in association with autoimmune diseases, malignancy, and medications, particularly penicillamine and captopril. Patients develop flaccid bullae, which rupture easily with application of pressure (referred to as a *positive Nikolsky sign*), on normal or slightly erythematous skin. The diagnosis of PV is made by identifying a loss of adhesion between keratinocytes (acantholysis) above the basal layer, resulting in an intraepidermal split. Bullous pemphigoid is also a self-limited autoimmune blistering disease characterized by tense, subepidermal bullae. Biopsies show subepidermal blisters rich with eosinophils (**A**). Neutrophil-rich infiltrates within dermal papillae (**C**) are seen in dermatitis herpetiformis, an intensely pruritic, papulovesicular skin disease characterized by lesions distributed over extensor surfaces. Hydropic degeneration of basal keratinocytes is more characteristic of lesions seen in DM or SLE. Eosinophilic necrosis of the epidermis (**E**) is seen with TEN or SJS, and patients present with painful erythematous macules with purpuric centers that tend to coalesce and ultimately lead to blisters and epidermal detachment over the entire body.

Pemphigus vulgaris

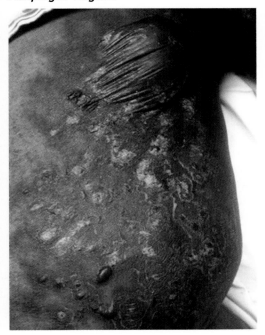

Pemphigus vulgaris (PV) is an autoimmune disease which causes chronic painful blistering of the skin. It is caused by antibodies against desmosome proteins (both desmoglein 1 and desmoglein 3), which results in loss of cohesion between keratinocytes in the epidermis. Extensive flaccid blisters and mucocutaneous erosions are typically seen. On histology, basal keratinocytes are usually still attached to the basement membrane, leading to the appearance and term *tombstoning*. PV is an intraepidermal process, whereas in bullous pemphigoid the detachment occurs between the epidermis and the dermis. Antidesmoglein autoantibodies can be visualized by direct immunofluorescence on a skin biopsy. The antibodies appear as IgG deposits along the desmosomes between epidermal cells.

- Definitive diagnosis via punch biopsy
- Treatment with corticosteroids and immunosuppressive drugs
- Acantholysis is the breaking apart of epidermal cells.
- Both cutaneous and mucosal lesions
- Flaccid bullae
- Positive Nikolsky sign

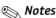 *Notes*

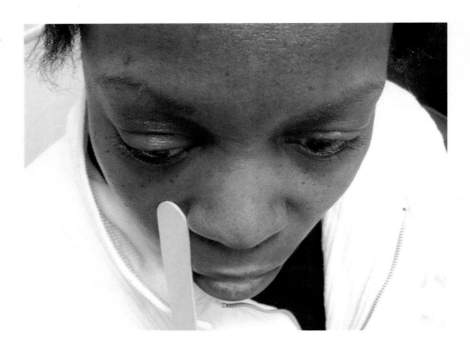

93. A 31-year-old woman with hyperthyroidism comes to the clinic for double vision. This occurs mainly when she tries to look up at objects. On physical examination, her eyes appear protruded, the right (see tongue blade) to a greater degree than the left. There is lid edema, lid retraction, and ophthalmoplegia on attempted upgaze. The patient is diagnosed with Graves ophthalmopathy. What symptom would require emergent treatment of her condition?

A. Afferent pupillary defect and slight loss of visual acuity
B. Diplopia in multiple gaze fields
C. Accompanying ptosis from myasthenia gravis (MG)
D. Corneal dryness
E. Coexisting bacterial sinusitis

94. A 36-year-old woman comes to clinic complaining of palpitations, excessive sweating, heat intolerance, nervousness, weight loss with increased appetite, difficulty sleeping, and infrequent periods (every 2-3 months). On exam, the patient's pulse is 115 bpm, and blood pressure is 130/85. She is diaphoretic and has notable exophthalmos with lid lag on downward gaze. She has pretibial skin thickening bilaterally. An electrocardiograph (ECG) reveals sinus tachycardia. Lab tests reveal low thyroid-stimulating hormone (TSH), high T_3, high T_4, and elevated thyroid-stimulating immunoglobulin. Radioactive iodine uptake is diffusely elevated throughout the thyroid gland. A β-blocker is prescribed. What is the best treatment for her underlying condition at this time?

A. Levothyroxine
B. Total thyroidectomy
C. Propylthiouracil
D. Radioactive iodine thyroid ablation

93. **The answer is A: Afferent pupillary defect and slight loss of visual acuity.** This patient has proptosis as a result of Graves disease. This hyperthyroid state occasionally causes engorgement (myxedema) of the extraocular muscles and forces the globe to protrude out. Successful management requires good control of the thyroid condition by an endocrinologist, but occasionally emergent intervention from an ophthalmologist is required. This situation involves compression of the optic nerve from the massively enlarged extraocular muscles. Early signs include an afferent pupillary defect, color vision impairment, and a slight decrease in visual acuity (**A**). If decompression is not achieved quickly, blindness may result.

94. **The answer is C: Propylthiouracil.** This patient is suffering from thyrotoxicosis due to effects of high levels of T_3 and T_4. Both the presence of thyroid-stimulating immunoglobulin and diffuse radioactive iodine uptake in the thyroid help confirm the diagnosis of Graves disease. Initial symptomatic therapy is with β-blockers to decrease tachycardia. First line therapy to achieve a euthyroid state is one of the thiocarbamide drugs (propylthiouracil, methimazole, carbimazole) to inhibit synthesis of thyroid hormone (**C**). This therapy is given for up to 2 years. Almost 50% of patients will continue to be euthyroid after thiocarbamide cessation. Other definitive therapies include thyroidectomy and radioactive iodine thyroid ablation. Levothyroxine is used in hypothyroid states.

Graves Proptosis

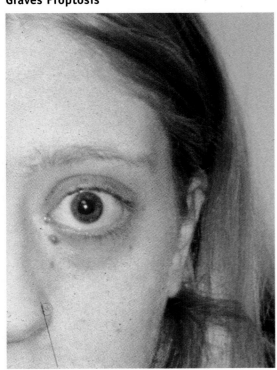

Graves disease denotes hyperthyroidism due to an autoimmune cause, and a small proportion of patients with this condition develop characteristic eye signs known as *Graves proptosis* (aka, *Graves ophthalmopathy, exophthalmos*). The proptosis is often asymmetric and may be accompanied by the cardinal signs and symptoms of lid retraction, corneal exposure, diplopia, gaze restriction, and visual loss.

- Protrusion of the globe results from orbital inflammation and engorgement of the extraocular muscles, especially the medial rectus and inferior rectus.
- Diplopia usually begins in the upper field of gaze but may progress to all fields of gaze when all extraocular muscles are involved.
- The optic nerve may be compressed and cause vision loss, which is a medical emergency.

✎ *Notes*
_____

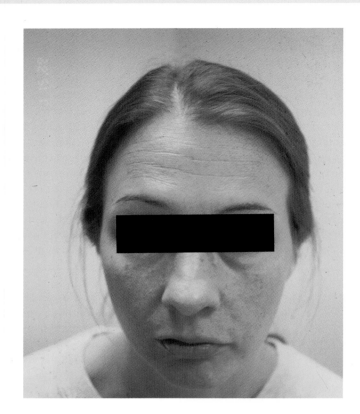

95. A 40-year-old woman presents with a 1-year history of easy bruising, oral ulcers, and a prominent rash over her cheeks and nasal bridge that seems to be more prominent after exposure to sunlight. Which of the following is not part of the diagnostic criteria for her disease?

A. Rash
B. Oral ulcers
C. Photosensitivity
D. Leukopenia
E. Hypercomplementemia

96. A 45-year-old woman presents with areas of hypopigmentation on the tragus area of both ears. She notes that over the past 2 years she has noticed red scaling patches in the same areas, but these always resolved after about a month. A review of systems is also significant for a history of joint pain and oral lesions occurring intermittently over the past 3 years. Which of the following is not a treatment that may be indicated for this patient's symptoms?

A. Topical sunscreens with SPF >30
B. Hydroxychloroquine
C. Thalidomide
D. Intralesional triamcinolone acetonide
E. Topical metronidazole

95. The answer is E: **Hypercomplementemia** is not part of the diagnostic criteria for lupus. Often hypocomplementemia is present in active lupus. This patient presents with classic findings of lupus, including a malar rash (**A**). Lupus patients may also develop a discoid rash, which appears as erythematous, raised patches with adherent keratotic scaling and follicular plugging. Oral ulcers (**B**) or nasopharyngeal ulceration may be present in lupus and are usually painless. Photosensitivity (**C**), arthritis, and serositis are also diagnostic criteria for lupus. Laboratory markers include proteinuria, leukopenia (**D**), lymphopenia, anemia, and thrombocytopenia.

96. The answer is E: **Topical metronidazole.** This patient is presenting with atrophy of the epidermis secondary to chronic cutaneous lupus, previously termed *discoid lupus.* Inflammation from the lesion destroys pigment, resulting in the hypopigmented area depicted in the image below. The patient also notes symptoms of systemic lupus, such as joint pain (occurs in over 90% of patients and is often the earliest manifestation of lupus) and oral ulcers. All of the above choices are potential treatments for discoid or systemic lupus except for (**E**) topical metronidazole, which is a treatment for rosacea and has no role in the treatment of discoid lupus. (**A**) Sunscreen with SPF >30 is recommended to prevent cutaneous symptoms. (**B**) An antimalarial, hydroxychloroquine, is often effective to treat the systemic and cutaneous manifestations of lupus. (**C**) Thalidomide is an effective treatment for discoid lupus in some patients. (**D**) Triamcinolone acetonide given intralesionally may be useful for smaller lesions, especially when steroids prove ineffective.

Lupus (Malar Rash)

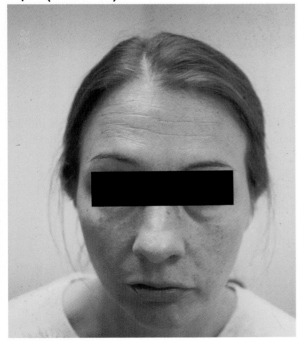

The *malar rash of lupus,* also called the *butterfly rash,* is one of the classic presentations of SLE. It is characterized by a flat or raised erythematous rash over the cheeks and bridge of the nose that spares the nasolabial folds and tends to occur after UV exposure. A malar rash can be present in diseases other than lupus, so a detailed history is very important. SLE is a chronic inflammatory disease that can affect the skin, joints, kidneys, lungs, nervous system, serous membranes, and/or other organs of the body. Immunologic abnormalities are also a prominent feature of the disease, especially the production of a number of ANA.

- SLE is most common in women in their 20s and 30s.
- Autoantibodies that are routinely assayed for lupus are ANA, antiphospholipid antibodies, anti-dsDNA, and Sm antibodies.
- Over 80% of lupus patients will have cutaneous manifestations of the disease at some point during their lifetime.

✎ *Notes*

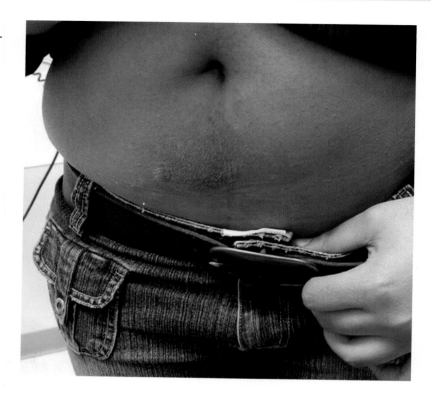

97. A 25-year-old woman presents to the office complaining of a rash on her lower abdomen. She states it started over a month ago as a small area of dry, itching skin. She had no relief with moisturizing cream and decided to seek treatment when the rash became larger. She has no other complaints and her past medical history is significant for mild, intermittent asthma. What is the best next step in the diagnosis and treatment of the rash?

A. Low-dose oral prednisone until the rash resolves
B. Allergen skin patch testing and topical diphenhydramine
C. Skin biopsy and referral to a dermatologist
D. Topical corticosteroids until the rash resolves
E. Careful history and avoidance of the offending agent

✎ *Notes*

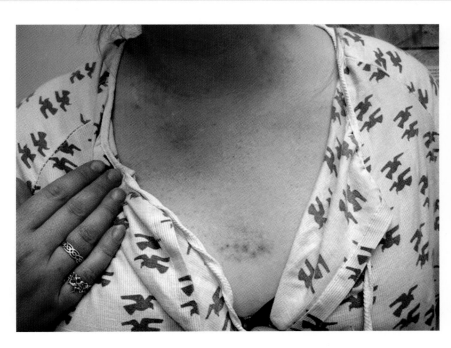

98. A 28-year-old woman complains of a rash on her neck. It has been present for 2 days and is intensely itchy. She attended a cocktail party 4 days ago, to which she wore a new necklace. Which of the following tests would confirm the cause of the lesion?

A. Potassium hydroxide preparation of scraping
B. Tzanck smear
C. Patch test
D. Culture
E. Complete blood count with differential

97. **The answer is E: Careful history and avoidance of the offending agent.** This patient is suffering from allergic contact dermatitis, a delayed-type hypersensitivity reaction to an exogenous agent, which in this case, is the patient's belt. Lesions often appear in the distribution of the contact. The best approach is to identify the allergen through a careful history and advise the patient to avoid contact with it (**E**). The immune reaction occurs in an individual who is genetically susceptible and has been previously sensitized by contact with the agent. The skin is pruritic and appears eczematous, with scaly, edematous patches and possibly weeping vesicles. Lichenification can occur with chronic exposure. Topical corticosteroids twice daily for 2-3 weeks can be used if the rash does not resolve with removal of the offending agent (**D**). Oral corticosteroids should only be used in severe cases and must be slowly tapered over more than 3 weeks to decrease the risk of rebound reactions (**A**). Skin patch testing should be used in cases where treatment fails (**B**). Allergic contact dermatitis is a clinical diagnosis, and skin biopsy is generally not warranted (**C**).

98. **The answer is C: Patch test.** The appearance of the lesion and history are consistent with allergic contact dermatitis. This patient's necklace was made of nickel, a common cause of this reaction. Contact dermatitis is diagnosed clinically, but after the lesion has been treated, sensitivity to the suspected allergen can be confirmed with a patch test (**C**). Atopic dermatitis and herpes zoster are also diagnosed clinically; however, eosinophilia may be seen in atopic dermatitis (**E**), and Tzanck smear (**B**) will show multinucleated giant cells in herpes simplex and varicella-zoster virus infections. In cases of cellulitis, culture (**D**) may be important for determining drug sensitivity. Potassium hydroxide preparation of scrapings can be used to diagnose fungal infections, such as tinea corporis and onychomycosis (**A**).

Allergic Contact Dermatitis

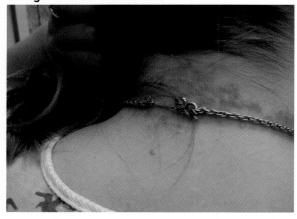

Allergic contact dermatitis is a delayed-type hypersensitivity reaction to an allergen to which a patient has been previously sensitized. Hands, feet, eyelids, and lips are common sites for contact dermatitis, since they often come in contact with the environment. Common allergens are contained in plants (poison ivy, poison oak), topical medications (neomycin, bacitracin, sulfonamides), jewelry (nickel), antiseptics (thimerosal), chemicals (formaldehyde), tree oils or perfumes, occupational exposures (chromium, cobalt), and rubber products (latex gloves).

- Allergic contact dermatitis may present acutely after allergen exposure and initial sensitization or after exposure in a previously sensitized individual.
- Acute phase is characterized by the development of erythematous, indurated, scaly plaques.
- Severe cases may demonstrate vesiculation and bullae.
- Lesions often mimic the pattern of exposure to the allergen.
- Treatment involves removal of the offending agent and topical or oral steroids and/or antihistamines in severe cases.

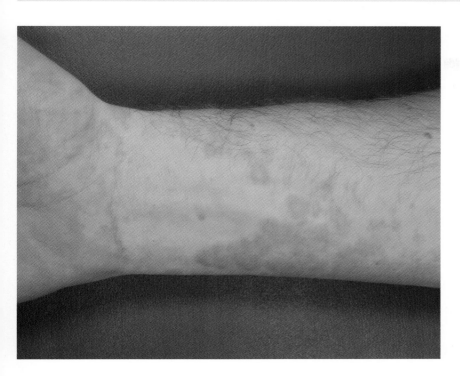

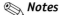
Notes _____

99. A 24-year-old man comes to the clinic complaining of a rash on his arms, hands, and feet. The rash developed yesterday and is pruritic. He also complains of myalgias, headache, and a painful rash in his genital region. He has been sexually active with four partners this year and only occasionally wears a condom. On physical exam, a maculopapular rash with target lesions is present on the forearms and palms. The genital rash is present at the base of the penis and consists of multiple vesicles on an erythematous base. A Tzanck smear reveals multinucleated giant cells, and the laboratory confirms detection of HSV-2 DNA by polymerase chain reaction. What is the best ongoing therapy for this patient?

A. Valacyclovir 500 mg once daily indefinitely

B. Hospitalization and admission to the burn unit

C. IV acyclovir 5 mg/kg q8h for 5 days and topical benadryl

D. Valacyclovir 1 g bid for 7-14 days, followed by valacyclovir 500 mg daily indefinitely

E. Oral prednisone 100 mg bid until resolution of the rash on the extremities and valacyclovir 1 g bid for 7-14 days

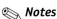

Notes

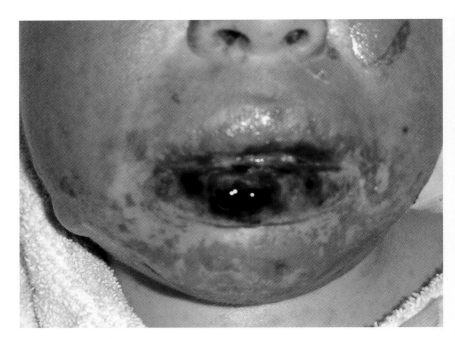

100. A 19-year-old woman comes in for a 1-week follow-up visit after being started on a course of amoxicillin for acute otitis media. The patient complains of fever to 102° F and a blistering rash around her mouth and hands that started 2 days ago. After the rash appeared, she discontinued antibiotic treatment. She has no fever today and is tolerating food and fluids. On physical exam, she is afebrile and her other vital signs are within normal limits. She has conjunctival hyperemia and red, coalescing macules and bullae on her face and hands. There is evidence of perioral epidermal necrosis and slight buccal mucosa desquamation. The lesions on the hands and face are positive for Nikolsky sign. Cultures are sent on blood, lesional fluid, and stool. What is the next best step in the management of this patient?

A. IV vancomycin 40 mg/kg/d for 2 days
B. Hospitalization and admission to the burn unit
C. IV acyclovir 5 mg/kg q8h for 5 days
D. Supportive care with hydration and close observation
E. Oral prednisone 50 mg/d for 7 days

99. The answer is D: Valacyclovir 1 g bid for 7-14 days, followed by valacyclovir 500 mg daily indefinitely. This patient is experiencing EM minor (now called *herpes-associated erythema multiforme* [HAEM]) which is characterized clinically by an acute inflammatory skin reaction consisting of symmetric maculopapular eruptions on the extremities, palms, and soles and classic "target" lesions. The mucous membranes of the mouth may be involved as well. The most common cause is HSV infection. Treatment of HAEM is generally not indicated unless the patient is unable to eat or the eye is involved. The patient should be treated for the acute HSV-2 genital lesions and then maintained on anti-HSV medication (such as valacyclovir) indefinitely to prevent recurrences of both rashes and decrease transmission of HSV (**D**).

100. The answer is D: Supportive care with hydration and close observation. This patient has SJS with amoxicillin as the trigger. A prodromal syndrome of fever and ocular and oral irritation usually precedes the skin rash of target lesions or erythematous macules/papules upon which bullae form on palms and soles, trunk, neck, proximal upper extremities, and face. Then the epidermis necrotizes and desquamates. SJS bullae usually form on at least two mucous membranes (conjunctivae, nares, mouth, anus, vagina, or urethral opening). This patient presented with classic ulcerative stomatitis and inflamed conjunctivae. Special care must be given to the conjunctivae, as ocular bullae and scarring can cause blindness. An ophthalmologist should follow these patients. The most appropriate care to be given at this time is supportive care (**D**). Triggers (allopurinol, antibiotics, anticonvulsants, and NSAIDs) must be discontinued. Since less than 6% of this patient's body surface area (BSA) is affected, there is no need to transfer her to a specialized burn unit at this time. She should, however, be given adequate hydration and nutrition, monitored for electrolyte disturbances and anemia, and reevaluated for percent BSA skin loss. Prophylactic antibiotic treatment is not used, and antiviral medication is not indicated (**A, C**). Although both glucocorticoids and intravenous immunoglobulin (IVIG) can be used, their efficacy has not been substantially proven (**E**). Both are reserved for more severe SJS and TEN.

Erythema Multiforme

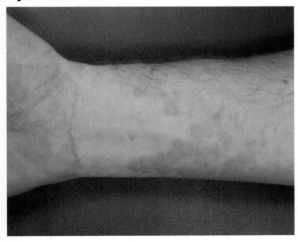

Erythema multiforme (EM) is an acute inflammatory skin disease that is divided clinically into major and minor types based on clinical findings. EM major favors the trunk, while EM minor affects the extensor surfaces, palms, soles, and mucous membranes. The lesions may be macular, papular, urticarial, bullous, or purpuric. EM minor is characterized by target lesions, which have a clear center and concentric, erythematous rings. Its course is often benign but frequently recurrent. The diagnosis is clinical. Treatment is reserved for severe cases with high BSA involvement, ocular manifestations, or oral mucosal involvement. Moderate to high-dose prednisone can be used as well as IVIG. Patients with severe EM major (>25–30% BSA) should be treated in a burn unit.

- The most common cause of EM minor is HSV infection (HAEM), and recurrences can be prevented by continued use of anti-HSV medication, such as valacyclovir or acyclovir.
- The most common cause of EM major in adults is drug-reactions (subtypes: SJS <10% BSA skin loss; TEN >30% BSA skin loss; overlap between 10% and 30% BSA skin loss in SJS and TEN).
- The clinical course has frequent recurrences, with frequency and severity tending to decrease spontaneously over 2 years or longer.

✎ *Notes*

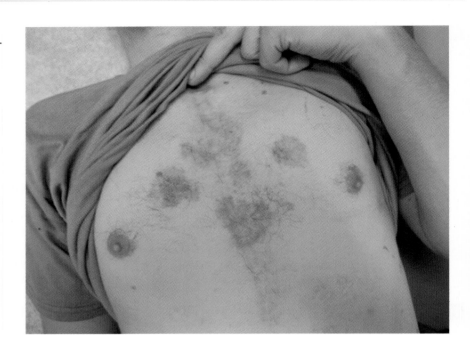

101. A 24-year-old man comes into the clinic during winter with a pruritic rash on his chest and leg for 3 weeks. He noticed dry, scaly, itchy, red areas on his chest that became inflamed and larger with scratching. He complains of itching and burning, which he admits have lessened in intensity since the rash first appeared. On physical exam, several erythematous, coin-shaped lesions, 2-4 cm in diameter, are noted on the chest and right popliteal fossa. The lesions are erythematous with mild thickening and undefined borders. Which of the following is/are the first-line treatment option(s)?

A. Avoiding irritants
B. Topical emollients
C. Antihistamine
D. Topical triamcinolone cream
E. All of the above

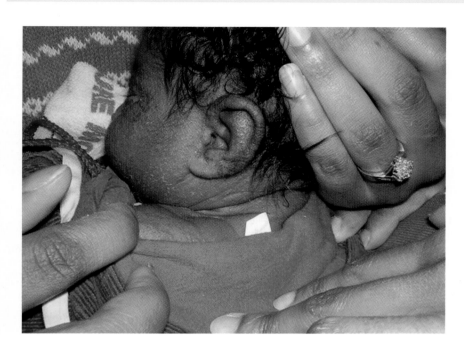

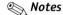

102. A mother brings her 1-month-old infant into the clinic with a new, red, flaky rash on her forehead, cheeks, ears, and scalp. On physical exam, greasy scaling and erythematous patches are noted on the patient's upper cheeks, forehead, ears, and scalp with particularly thick white scaling on the vertex of the scalp. Which of the following statements is/are true regarding this patient's diagnosis?

A. Treated with topical ketoconazole
B. Treated with selenium sulfide shampoo
C. Fungi of *Malassezia (Pityrosporum)* genus is a factor in the inflammatory process.
D. Infantile seborrheic dermatitis disappears in the first year of life.
E. All of the above

101. **The answer is E: All of the above.** This patient has nummular (discoid) eczema with atopic dermatitis in a subacute stage (dry, red, scaly, itchy). These lesions often appear on the dorsal surface of hands or extensor surfaces of forearms and legs. The key to treatment is removing known irritants (hot showers, excessive washing, drying, scratching) and allergens. Keeping the lesions moist with topical emollients decreases irritation and inflammation. Antihistamines are sometimes needed to decrease intense itching that can elicit scratching, particularly during sleep. Although oral steroids are indicated in some acute stages in order to penetrate eczematous vesicles, topical steroids (triamcinolone) efficiently speed resolution of these dry, subacute lesions. Although not as rapid-acting as steroids, the immunosuppressives tacrolimus and pimecrolimus prevent production of cytokines, which can be useful in controlling inflammation. So all of these treatments (**E**) can be used to treat eczema, which resolves or becomes chronic in nature.

102. **The answer is E: All of the above.** The patient is diagnosed with seborrheic dermatitis, commonly referred to in infants as *cradle cap*. Seborrheic dermatitis can be treated with the antifungal ketoconazole, topical low-potency steroids for inflammation, and/or antiseborrheic shampoos (selenium sulfide) for the scaling. *Malassezia* requires fat to survive and is present in dermal regions of highly concentrated sebaceous glands where seborrheic dermatitis appears. Infantile seborrheic dermatitis is most prevalent in the first 3 months of life and usually dissipates by 1 year of age. Application of topical baby oils followed by combing the hair with a fine-toothed comb can be used to remove large scales from the scalp. So all of these treatments (**E**) can be used to treat seborrheic dermatitis.

Dermatitis

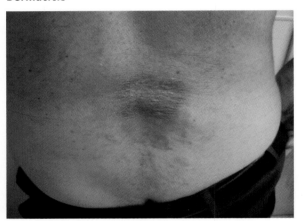

The term *dermatitis* encompasses a variety of skin conditions that may present in different ways. Some cases present with acute edema, erythema, and oozing with crusting; some with mild erythema alone; and others with lichenification, which is the result of chronic irritation. Histologically, the many forms of dermatitis are difficult to distinguish, but known causes and the natural history of lesions helps to categorize the conditions. These types include but are not limited to atopic dermatitis, nummular eczema, primary irritant contact dermatitis, allergic contact dermatitis, seborrheic dermatitis, and dry-skin dermatitis (xerosis).

- Atopic dermatitis is chronic superficial inflammation of skin. It may have three clinical phases (infantile eczema, childhood or flexural eczema, adolescent eczema). Treatment consists of avoiding irritants, keeping the skin moist, and topical corticosteroids or immunosuppressive agents.
- Nummular eczema presents with numerous symmetric, coin-shaped patches of dermatitis on the extremities. Treatment is similar to atopic dermatitis.
- Primary irritant contact dermatitis appears within hours of contact, peaks at 24 hours, and then disappears. The most common form is diaper dermatitis, caused by prolonged contact of the skin with urine and feces. Treatment is to increase the frequency of diaper changes and wash with water after a bowel movement.
- Allergic contact dermatitis is a delayed-type hypersensitivity reaction to offending agent. There is delayed onset around 18 hours, which then peaks at 48-72 hours and may last as long as 2-3 weeks even after cessation of contact with the allergen. Nickel, latex, and poison ivy are very common causes of allergic contact dermatitis. Allergic contact dermatitis commonly causes blister formation with oozing and crusting, often in the pattern of allergen exposure. Treatment mainly involves avoidance of triggers.
- Seborrheic dermatitis is erythematous, scaly dermatitis and high sebum production in areas containing a high density of sebaceous glands (face, scalp, and perineum). First-line treatment involves topical antifungal agents (such as ketoconazole); resistant cases can be treated with topical corticosteroids.
- Dry-skin dermatitis (xerosis) presents with large cracked scales with erythematous borders and occurs in arid environments. Treatment is aimed at increasing water content of skin by minimizing bathing, avoiding soaps, and frequently using emollients.

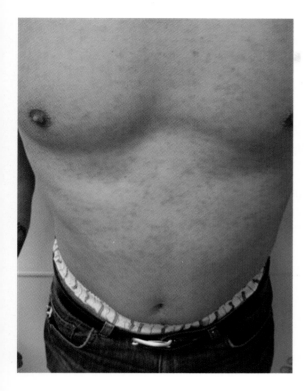

103. A 32-year-old man presents with a red-brown maculopapular rash over his trunk and extremities. The rash is present over his palms and soles. He has had a fever and headache over the past week. He currently takes no medications and has never had an adverse reaction to medications. About a month ago, he remembers having a firm, painless skin ulceration on the shaft of his penis. He denies other skin lesions. What is the first line treatment for this patient?

A. One dose of IM benzathine penicillin G (2.4 million units)
B. IM benzathine penicillin G (2.4 million units) given once a week for 3 weeks
C. Doxycycline 100 mg bid for 2 weeks
D. One dose of azithromycin 2 g taken orally
E. Tetracycline 500 mg taken orally four times daily for 2 weeks

104. A 28-year-old man at the refugee clinic is concerned about a single, firm, non-itchy, painless skin ulceration with a clean base and sharp borders that has been on his penis for the past 3 weeks. He admits to having unprotected sex 2 months ago. If left untreated, what is the most likely long-term tertiary manifestation of this disease?

A. Infection involving the CNS, such as general paresis or tabes dorsalis
B. Syphilitic aortitis and possible aneurysm formation
C. Saddle nose deformation and Clutton joints
D. Soft, tumor-like balls of inflammation which may affect the skin, liver, and bone
E. Reddish-pink, non-itchy rash that occurs on the trunk, arms, palms, and soles

103. The answer is A: One dose of IM benzathine penicillin G (2.4 million units). This patient has a rash characteristic of secondary syphilis. Because he recalls having a primary lesion 1 month ago, the duration of illness is known. This patient should be treated with one dose of IM benzathine penicillin G 2.4 million units (A). One dose of IM penicillin G is given once weekly for 3 weeks (B) to treat tertiary syphilis or secondary syphilis that has been present for more than 1 year. If the patient is penicillin allergic, doxycycline 100 mg bid for 2 weeks (C) or tetracycline 500 mg four times daily for 2 weeks (E) can be used as alternatives. There is limited data to support a one-time dose of azithromycin 2 g (D), and this is not first-line treatment.

104. The answer is D: Soft, tumor-like balls of inflammation which may affect the skin, liver, and bone. This patient presents with classic symptoms of primary syphilis. If left untreated, this will progress to secondary syphilis 4-10 weeks later, manifesting as a non-itchy red rash on the trunk and extremities, including the palms and soles (D). This rash will likely resolve in 3-6 weeks. Tertiary syphilis is the long-term complication that may occur due to syphilis and can be divided into three forms: late neurosyphilis (A) affects 6.5%, gummatous syphilis affects the majority (15%), and cardiovascular syphilis (10%). Saddle nose deformation and Clutton joints (C) are manifestations of congenital syphilis.

Syphilis (Chancre and Secondary)

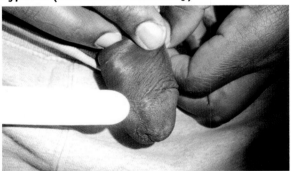

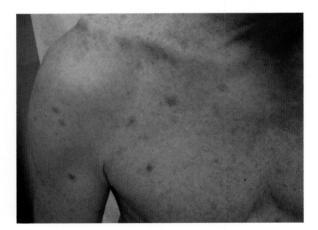

Syphilis is a sexually transmitted disease caused by the spirochete *Treponema pallidum*. Syphilis can generally be treated with antibiotics, including penicillin. If untreated, syphilis can damage the heart, aorta, bones, eyes, and brain. Primary syphilis is typically acquired by direct sexual contact. Approximately 2–6 weeks after the initial exposure, a skin lesion appears at the point of contact, which is usually the genitalia. This lesion, called a *chancre,* is a firm, painless skin ulceration. The lesion may persist for 4-6 weeks and usually heals spontaneously. Secondary syphilis occurs 1-6 months after the primary infection (average 6-8 weeks). There are many manifestations of secondary syphilis. A red or brown maculopapular rash may develop over the trunk and extremities and may involved the palms and soles. Other symptoms may include fever, malaise, weight loss, headache, or enlarged lymph nodes. Secondary syphilis also commonly involves the mucous membranes. Latent syphilis is present when there is serologic evidence of syphilis, but the patient does not have physical signs of the disease. Late or tertiary syphilis involves the cardiovascular system, CNS, and ocular system. Gummatous lesions may involve the skin, bones, or viscera.

- Serologic screening tests include RPR and venereal disease research laboratory (VDRL). All positive tests should be confirmed with treponemal antibody test (FTA-ABS).
- Treatment for early disease (primary and secondary for less than 1 year) is one dose benzathine penicillin G. For late disease, benzathine penicillin G is given once a week for 3 weeks.
- Darkfield microscopic examination can be used to visualize spirochetes.

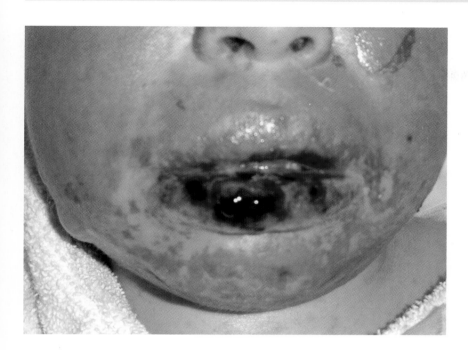

✎ **Notes** _____

105. A 30-year-old woman presents with fever and painful mucocutaneous lesions. She notes that she has no medical conditions. Her primary care doctor started her on a sulfa drug for a bacterial infection 4 days ago. You note sloughing of the epidermis on physical exam. What is the most appropriate treatment?

A. Stop sulfonamide antibiotic immediately
B. Administer analgesics
C. Start IV fluids
D. Initiate NG or parenteral feeding
E. All of the above

106. A 28-year-old woman with a history of epilepsy presents to your office complaining of fever, sore throat, and fatigue for 5 days' duration. She comes to you today because she began to notice ulcers in her mouth and lips (shown above). These ulcers are extremely painful, and she is beginning to have difficulty eating and drinking. You stop the mediation and start supportive therapy. Which of the following findings would support a diagnosis of SJS?

A. More than 30% BSA epidermal detachment
B. Involvement of the hair-bearing scalp
C. Well-demarcated plaques of hypopigmentation that are cool to the touch
D. Presence of Nikolsky sign

105. The answer is E: All of the above. This woman is suffering a severe drug hypersensitivity reaction. The involvement of skin and mucous membranes is consistent with SJS. All of the above (E) are necessary treatment steps for SJS. All medications should be stopped immediately (A), especially those known to cause SJS reactions (such as sulfonamides, amoxicillin, penicillin, and allopurinol). Supportive care, such as analgesics (B), IV fluids (C) and NG or parenteral feeding (D), should also be initiated.

106. The answer is D: Well-demarcated plaques of hypopigmentation that are cool to the touch. Lamotrigine is traditionally known to lead to SJS. Other medications include sulfonamides, penicillins, phenytoin, and barbiturates. Presence of Nikolsky sign is common in SJS and often helps to differentiate the condition from fixed drug eruptions (D). Fixed drug eruptions appear, 7-10 days after exposure, involve a defined area of hypopigmentation, and are rarely hot to the touch. Involvement of 30% or more of the skin is suggestive of TEN. Involvement of the hair-bearing scalp is rare in SJS (B).

Stevens-Johnson Syndrome (SJS)

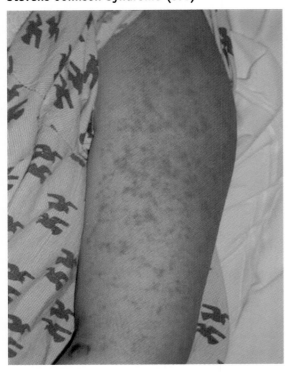

Stevens-Johnson syndrome (SJS) is a life-threatening condition characterized by fever and mucocutaneous lesions leading to necrosis and sloughing of the epidermis. The syndrome affects the skin and the mucous membranes and is thought to be a hypersensitivity complex. SJS is less severe than TEN in that a lesser percent of the body surface is involved (defined as less than 10% to 30% of the body surface is involved). This syndrome is most commonly triggered by medications, but it can also be caused by infections, cancers, or may be idiopathic. SJS is an emergency, and all medications should be immediately discontinued, particularly those known to cause SJS reactions. Initially treatment is similar to that for patients with thermal burns (IV fluids, NG or parenteral feeding, analgesics, etc).

- Affects skin and mucous membranes
- Mucous membranes are affected in 92% to 100% of patients.
- Stop medications immediately.
- Treat with supportive measures

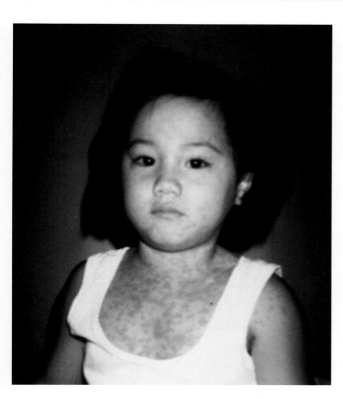

107. A 7-year-old girl is brought to the pediatrician by her mother. She notes that the patient has been quite ill with a fever, cough, and runny nose for the past 5 days. She noticed today that a rash was developing on her head and face. Her mother also noticed small white spots on her oral mucosa while she was helping her brush her teeth a couple of days ago. On physical examination, you note that the girl has conjunctivitis and a maculopapular rash over her upper body. What is the cause of this girl's illness?

A. Rubella virus
B. HHV-6
C. Varicella-zoster virus
D. Paramyxovirus
E. Parvovirus B19

✎ *Notes*

_____

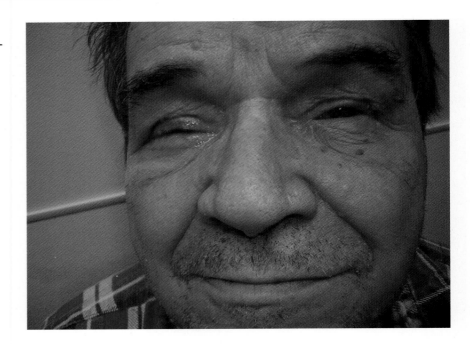

108. A 65-year-old man born in Poland with an unknown medical history presents for the first time to his primary care physician in Arizona complaining of a 3-day history of cough, fever of 101°-103° F, runny nose, and "pink eye." On physical exam, the patient's right conjunctiva is injected, and his eyelid is encrusted with yellow mucus. He also has rhinorrhea and on oral exam is found to have white lesions with an erythematous halo on his buccal mucosa but no tonsilar erythema or edema. Rapid strep, influenza, and monospot tests are negative. On further questioning, the patient had recently been exposed his granddaughter who he reports had a "rash" on her face and chest. What is the most likely diagnosis of this patient's constellation of symptoms?

A. Influenza
B. Scarlet fever
C. Measles
D. Infectious mononucleosis
E. Toxoplasmosis

107. **The answer is D: Paramyxovirus.** This girl is presenting with measles (rubeola) which is caused by a paramyxovirus (**D**). Classic symptoms include fever, cough, coryza, and conjunctivitis. In addition, this mother noticed white spots on the girl's buccal mucosa, possibly representing Koplik spots, which are pathognomonic for the disease and are seen before the rash. The typical rash of measles is erythematous and maculopapular, starting on the head and spreading to the body. Rubella virus (**A**) causes lymphadenopathy and an erythematous rash that starts on the face and spreads distally. In contrast to measles, children with rubella often are not as ill and do not present with cough, coryza, conjunctivitis, or Koplik spots. HHV-6 causes roseola infection. These patients present with an acute onset of a high fever, which lasts 3-4 days. As the fever breaks, a maculopapular rash starts on the trunk before spreading to the face and extremities. Varicella (**C**) causes generalized pruritic vesicular lesions that are often visualized at different stages of healing. Parvovirus B19 (**E**) causes fifth disease (erythema infectiosum). Fifth disease causes a "slapped-cheek" erythematous rash. A maculopapular, erythematous rash can be seen, starting on the arms and spreading to the legs and trunk.

108. **The answer is C: Measles.** Given this patient's signs and symptoms, he is most likely presenting with a case of adult-onset measles (**C**), caused by a paramyxovirus infection. Measles begin with a 2- to 4-day respiratory prodrome of malaise, cough, coryza, conjunctivitis, rhinorrhea, and high fevers. Often patients will also demonstrate Koplik spots (1- to 2-mm, blue-white spots on a red background) on the buccal mucosa just before the onset of an erythematous, nonpruritic, maculopapular rash beginning on the head and spreading down the trunk and arms to include the palms and soles. Although this disease is rare in the United States and was declared eliminated in 2002, recent outbreaks are becoming increasingly common. In 2008, 140 confirmed cases were reported to the CDC, and 25% of those were found in adults. Twenty-two of the 140 total cases were reported in Arizona. These outbreaks primarily affected those who had not been vaccinated with the measles, mumps, and rubella (MMR) vaccine, due either to cases imported from other countries or to a recent resistance of some parents to vaccinate their children due to scientifically unfounded fears of an association between the vaccine and autism. Because this patient was born outside of the United States, it is likely that he never received the MMR vaccine and thus was susceptible to becoming infected from his grandchild. Influenza (**A**) may present with a cough, fever, and rhinorrhea but generally does not cause conjunctivitis. Given this patient's negative rapid flu test, this is not the most likely diagnosis. Scarlet fever (**B**) presents as a "sandpapery" rash occurring on the neck and chest following infection with group A streptococci. The patient's constellation of symptoms are not seen with group A strep infections, and given his negative rapid strep test, this is not the diagnosis. Infectious mononucleosis (**D**) is caused by the EBV. It may present with fever, sore throat, malaise, anorexia, and myalgia, along with the physical findings of lymphadenopathy, splenomegaly, and, less commonly, a maculopapular rash. Although the virus may occasionally cause exudative pharyngitis or tonsillitis, Koplik spots are not seen. The virus does have the potential to cause conjunctival hemorrhage in the eye but does not present with conjunctivitis like that seen in measles patients. Toxoplasmosis (**E**) in immunocompetent patients presents with few, if any, symptoms. The protozoan *Toxoplasma gondii* may infrequently lead to mild lymphadenopathy, low-grade fevers, and sore throat. Chorioretinitis may result from reactivation of congenital toxoplasmosis, but conjunctivitis is not seen.

Measles

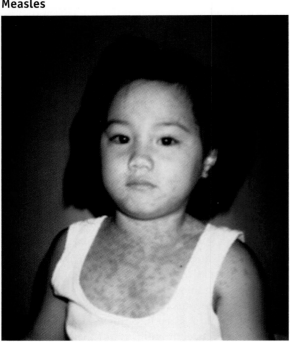

Measles, also called *rubeola,* is an infection of the respiratory system caused by a paramyxovirus. The viral infection produces an erythematous maculopapular rash. The rash erupts 5 days after onset of prodromal symptoms. Typically the rash begins on the head and then spreads to the body, lasting 4-5 days. Koplik spots are white spots on the buccal mucosa, which resolve prior to the appearance of the rash. Koplik spots are pathognomonic for the disease when they are seen. Typical associated symptoms include fever and the Three Cs (cough, coryza, conjunctivitis). Common complications include otitis media, pneumonia, and laryngotracheitis. A rare complication of measles is subacute sclerosing panencephalitis.

- Diagnosis: fever and the Three Cs (cough, coryza, conjunctivitis)
- Children are vaccinated for measles as part of the MMR vaccine.
- Spread through respiratory fluids, either via direct contact or through aerosol transmission

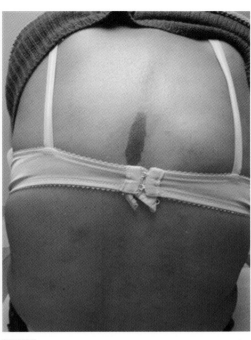

109. A 26-year-old woman has had the above large, flat lesion on her back since birth. She is concerned about the risk of developing melanoma, from which a colleague at work just died. She would like to know if the lesion should be removed. She has fewer than 20 nevomelanocytic nevi on her body, and there is no history of skin cancer in her family. How should she be counseled regarding this lesion?

A. There is a high risk of progression to melanoma, and the lesion should be removed.
B. There is a mild risk of progression to melanoma, so the lesion should be examined every 6 months.
C. The lesion is benign, and excision can cause disfiguration; therefore, excision is not advisable.
D. The lesion must be biopsied before a treatment decision can be made.
E. The lesion is malignant and has a poor prognosis.

110. A 20-year-old woman with blue eyes presents to the office for an annual visit. She has no complaints and no significant past medical history. She spends her summers away from college at the beach, where she works as a swimming teacher. Her family history is significant for her maternal grandmother having basal cell carcinoma of her nose. With further questioning, she admits to occasional sunburns. Total body skin exam reveals multiple melanocytic nevi on her trunk and arms, numbering over 50, which she states have been there for some time. None of the nevi measure over 5 mm in diameter. The nevi all have a round or oval shape with sharp borders and light brown pigmentation. Which of the following statements about this patient is true?

A. The development of benign nevi is stimulated by UV radiation exposure.
B. The number of benign nevi on this patient places her at higher risk for developing melanoma.
C. Growth alone may not be sufficient reason to excise a nevus.
D. Obtaining baseline photographic documentation of this patient's nevi can help guide future treatment strategies.
E. All of the above

109. **The answer is C: The lesion is benign, and excision can cause disfiguration; therefore, excision is not advisable.** This is a congenital nevus, which is a benign proliferation of normal skin constituents. It is present from birth and arises from cells deep in the subcutaneous fat; therefore, excision is difficult and can cause significant disfiguration (**C**). There is a low risk of progression to malignancy (**A, B, E**). She has fewer than 50 nevi and no family history of skin cancer; therefore, she is not at increased risk of developing melanoma. This is a clinical diagnosis, and biopsy is not necessary (**D**).

110. **The answer is E: All of the above.** All of the above statements are correct (**E**). This patient is a fair-eyed individual who has a considerable amount of sun exposure due to her occupation and has had sun damage as evidenced by her history of sunburns. Her skin findings are consistent with the presence of multiple benign nevi, also known as *acquired melanocytic nevi*. This patient is at risk for subsequent development of melanoma and non-melanoma skin cancer because of her high cumulative UV radiation exposure and family history of cutaneous malignancy, as well as the number of benign nevi present on her skin (>50). Thus, she should be assessed with total body skin examinations during her annual office visit. Photographic documentation of her findings can help track the skin findings over time. Because benign nevi are often still in development at her age, some can be expected to grow and may not necessarily need excision in the absence of other concerning features, which may include irregular and ill-defined borders, eccentric pigment patterns, and rapid growth. Dermatoscopy can aid in tracking lesions over time and making decisions on treatment strategies.

Benign Nevus

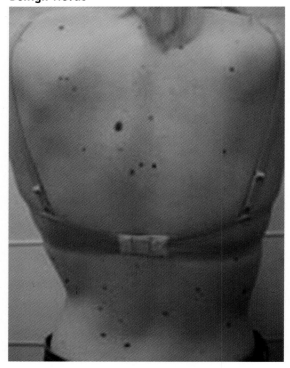

A *benign nevus* develops slowly after birth, usually during childhood or young adulthood, and grows symmetrically before stabilizing at a certain size. Some may regress after a period of time. Environmental exposure to UV radiation seems to be the inciting factor for the development of benign nevi. Genetic factors play a role as well, and there is an association with pale skin, blue or green eyes, blond or light-brown hair, and a tendency to sunburn.

- Develop after birth and are typically smaller than 5 mm
- Flat or raised; symmetric, smooth, well-defined border; uniform pigmentation
- Higher lifetime risk of melanoma in patients with more than 50 benign nevi
- Excision is difficult and disfiguring and, therefore, usually not performed.

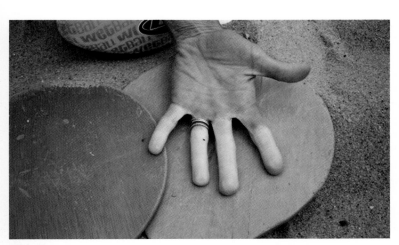

111. The 45-year-old woman in the picture above presents to your office complaining of blanching of her fingers, extending from the tips to various levels of the digits with sparing of the thumb whenever she is cold or stressed out. She is otherwise healthy and has a negative review of systems. Which of the following statements are true in regard to her condition?

A. It is usually seen in older male patients.
B. She is at high risk for developing an autoimmune disease, even if she does not develop any additional symptoms for more than 2 years.
C. Drug therapy using calcium channel blockers (CCBs) can be used for severe cases.
D. Smoking cessation does not improve symptoms.
E. It is most commonly associated with ankylosing spondylitis.

112. A 35-year-old woman presents to your office complaining of pain and tingling in her fingers and toes. She recently took a trip to Quebec to ice-climb and describes a particular episode where she noticed this pain and tingling and removed her gloves to find that her fingers had developed a startling blue hue and then turned white. You recommend that she avoid unnecessary cold environments and dress warmly, taking care to protect her trunk as well as her extremities. In addition, you recommend that she stop smoking, as tobacco can exacerbate constriction of her blood vessels. Despite her compliance, her symptoms persist. She returns to you desperate for a medication to help alleviate her symptoms. You prescribe a medication to reduce the frequency and severity of her attacks. Which of the following is the mechanism of action of the medication?

A. Block voltage-gated calcium channels in blood vessels, decreasing intracellular calcium, resulting in decreased contraction of the vascular smooth muscle and increase in arterial diameter
B. Block the conversion of angiotensin I to angiotensin II, thereby lowering arteriolar resistance and increasing venous capacity
C. Penetrate the vascular endothelium and cause nitrous oxide production, which activates cyclic guanosine monophosphate, ultimately leading to venodilation
D. Increase reabsorption of calcium in the distal convoluted tubule of the kidney and decrease sodium transport, leading to natriuresis and water loss
E. Reduce dopaminergic and adrenergic transmission in the peripheral nervous system, lowering blood pressure and sympathetic nervous system output

111. **The answer is C: Drug therapy using calcium channel blockers (CCBs) can be used for severe cases.** This patient has RP, an abnormal constriction of the blood vessels in response to cold, mental stress, or smoking. It is seen in 10%-20% of young women (**A**), and the sequence of color changes include pallor (white) with sharp demarcation as above, then cyanosis (blue) because of slow blood flow, followed by erythema (red) reflecting the reactive hyperemic phase. RP (secondary Raynaud) should be distinguished from Raynaud disease (primary Raynaud). RP is associated with scleroderma (most common, with 90% prevalence) (**E**), DM, mixed connective tissue disease, RA, SLE, Sjögren, cryoglobulinemia, and vasculitides like polyarteritis. Young female patients who have had RP alone for more than 2 years and have not developed any additional manifestations are at low risk for developing an autoimmune disease (**B**) and would have primary RD instead. Smoking cessation is mandatory due to the vasoconstrictive effects (**D**), and drug therapy using CCBs should be reserved for severe cases only (**C**).

112. **The answer is A: Block voltage-gated calcium channels in blood vessels, decreasing intracellular calcium, resulting in decreased contraction of the vascular smooth muscle and increase in arterial diameter.** CCBs such as nifedipine work by decreasing intracellular calcium, resulting in increased blood flow to ischemic extremities. These medications are commonly prescribed to treat severe RP. ACE inhibitors (**B**) and thiazide diuretics (**D**) are commonly used to treat hypertension and have little use in alleviating the symptoms associated with RP. Nitrates (**C**) and methyldopa (**E**) can be used to treat RP, but only in severe cases that are refractory to CCB treatment or where CCBs are otherwise contraindicated or poorly tolerated.

Raynaud Phenomenon

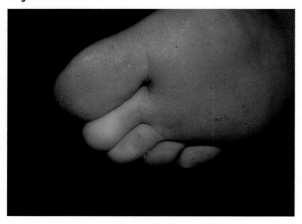

Raynaud phenomenon (RP) is a condition resulting in a series of discolorations of the fingers and/or the toes after exposure to changes in temperature. Skin discoloration occurs because an abnormal spasm of the blood vessels causes a decreased blood supply to the local tissues. Initially the digit(s) involved turns white because of the diminished blood supply. The digit(s) then turns blue because of prolonged lack of oxygen. Finally the blood vessels reopen, causing a local "flushing" phenomenon, which turns the digit(s) red.

- More common in women
- May be part of CREST syndrome
- CCBs for symptom control
- Most commonly found in fingers, toes, and other acral areas such as the nose and ears

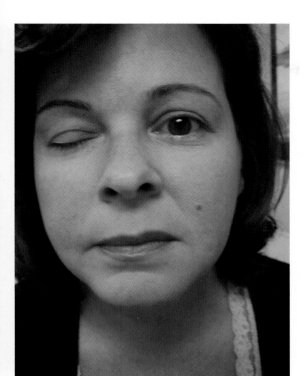

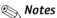

113. A 42-year-old woman presents with repeated episodes of a drooping right eyelid, which becomes more noticeable in the evenings. She states that she is in good health but has been experiencing transient episodes of eyelid drooping and double vision. She also has experienced intermittent difficulty with prolonged chewing and swallowing. What is the mechanism causing this patient's symptoms?

A. Antibodies to presynaptic voltage-dependent calcium channels
B. Antibodies to postsynaptic acetylcholine receptors
C. Toxin
D. Degeneration of motor neurons
E. Viral infection

114. A 32-year-old woman presents due to episodes of drooping of her right eyelid and blurry vision that seem to be worse later in the day. She has no significant medical or family history and takes no medications. Physical exam is significant for right-sided ptosis and diplopia as well as progressive weakness with prolonged arm abduction. A laboratory test shows the presence of anti–acetylcholine receptor (anti-AChR) antibodies in the patient's serum. All of the following additional screening tests would be indicated in this patient except?

A. CT scan of the anterior mediastinum
B. TSH and T_3/T_4 levels
C. ANA
D. Fine needle aspiration (FNA) of the thyroid
E. Rheumatoid factor

113. **The answer is B: Antibodies to postsynaptic acetylcholine receptors.** This patient is experiencing symptoms consistent with myasthenia gravis (MG), including transient ocular and bulbar muscle fatigue which worsens as the day progresses. MG is caused by antibodies to postsynaptic acetylcholine receptors (**B**). Antibodies to presynaptic voltage-dependent calcium channels (**A**) are found in Lambert-Eaton syndrome. The classic presentation of Lambert-Eaton syndrome includes proximal leg weakness, autonomic dysfunction, and ptosis, but rarely includes involvement of the bulbar muscles. Symptoms in Lambert-Eaton are worse in the morning and improve with exercise. Approximately half of Lambert-Eaton patients have cancer, usually of the small-cell lung type. A toxin-mediated process (**C**), such as botulism, may cause bulbar and eye muscle involvement. However, pupillary paralysis is common, and there is often rapid progression following ingestion of food contaminated by *Clostridium botulinum*. MG typically spares pupillary muscles. Degeneration of motor neurons (**D**), as seen in amyotrophic lateral sclerosis (ALS), typically does not produce ptosis or diplopia. ALS may be associated with bulbar muscle weakness. Patients have findings of upper motor neuron and lower motor neuron involvement. Bell palsy, which may be caused by a viral infection, causes facial palsy. The history of multiple transient episodes of ptosis makes Bell palsy less likely in this case.

114. **The answer is A: CT scan of the anterior mediastinum.** This patient presents with several of the signs and symptoms of MG, a condition caused by autoantibodies to postsynaptic acetylcholine receptors. The presence of anti-AChR antibodies in a patient's serum is diagnostic of this disease. Anti-AchR antibodies are detectable in the serum of close to 85% of myasthenic patients but in only about 50% of patients with weakness confined to the ocular muscles, which is seen earlier in the disease process. These patients have an increased incidence of several associated disorders. Seventy-five percent of patients exhibit thymic abnormalities, and many may exhibit enlargement of the thymus due to neoplastic changes, and therefore these patients should be screened with a CT scan of the anterior mediastinum (**A**). Hyperthyroidism may be seen in 3%-8% of patients and may exacerbate their weakness, so thyroid function tests (**B**) should be obtained in all patients with MG. There is also an association with other autoimmune disorders, and patients with MG should have blood tests for rheumatoid factor (**E**) and ANA (**C**). FNA (**D**) of the thyroid is not indicated for patients with MG.

Myasthenia Gravis

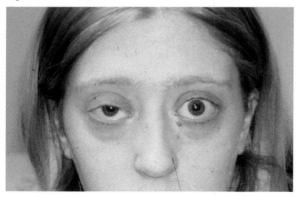

Myasthenia gravis (MG) is an autoimmune neuromuscular disease characterized by fluctuating weakness and fatigability in ocular, bulbar, limb, and respiratory muscles that increases with repeated use. Weakness is the result of T cell–dependent, antibody-mediated attack on postsynaptic acetylcholine receptors of the neuromuscular junction. Patients present with ptosis, ocular palsies, and proximal muscle weakness, which worsens as the day progresses.

- Physical exam, repetitive nerve stimulation test, and edrophonium (Tensilon) test can be performed if diagnosis is suspected. Tensilon is a short-acting cholinesterase inhibitor that allows for normal synaptic function in affected muscles.
- A more specific test to detect autoantibodies should be done to confirm diagnosis.
- Screen for thymomas with a chest CT.
- Treat medically with cholinesterase inhibitors (neostigmine) or immunosuppressants. Thymectomy may be indicated in some cases.
- During crisis, intubation may be needed for respiratory support, along with plasmapheresis.

References – Board Images

Fauci, A. S., Braunwald, E., Kasper, D. L., Hauser, S. L., Longo, D. L., Jameson, J. L., et al. (March 6, 2008). *Harrison's principles of internal medicine* (17th ed.). **McGraw-Hill Professional.**

Grimes, P. E., (1995, December). Melasma. Etiologic and therapeutic considerations, *Arch Dermatol*, *131*(12):1453–1457.

Hall, J. B., Schmidt, G. A., & Wood L. D. H. (July 2005). *Principles of critical care* (3rd ed.). **McGraw-Hill Professional**.

Higgins, S. P., Freemark, M., & Prose, N. S. (2008, September 15). Acanthosis nigricans: a practical approach to evaluation and management. *Dermatol Online J*, *14*(9), 2.

Knoop, K. J., Stack, L. B., Storrow, A. B., & Thurman, R. J. (July 2002). *The Atlas of emergency medicine* (3rd ed.). **McGraw-Hill Professional**.

McPhee, S. J., & Papadakis, M. A. (2011). Lange Medical Books/McGraw-Hill, 2010.

Rutter, M. 2005. Incidence of autism spectrum disorders: changes over time and their meaning, *Acta Paediatr 94*(1):2–15.

Tintinalli, J. E., Stapczynski, J. S., Cline, D. M., Ma, O. J., Cydulka, R. K., & Meckler, G. D. (October 14, 2003). *Tintinalli's Emergency medicine: A comprehensive study guide* (7th ed.). **McGraw-Hill Professional**.

Wolff, K., Goldsmith, L. A., Katz, S. I., Gilchrest, B., Paller, A. S., & Leffell, D. J. (October 17, 2007). Thomas Brenn, Neoplasms of subcutaneous fat. In *Fitzpatrick's Dermatology in general medicine* (7th ed.). **McGraw-Hill Professional**.

Wolff, K., & Johnson, R. A. (2009). *Fitzpatrick's Color atlas and synopsis of clinical dermatology*, (6th ed.). **New York**: McGraw Hill.

Section II
CARDIOLOGY

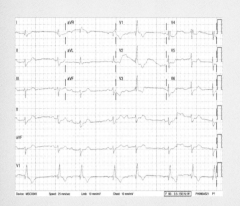
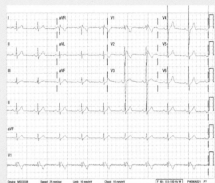
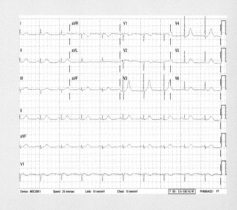

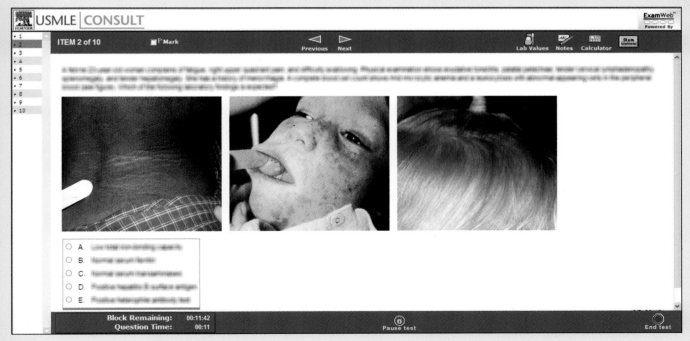

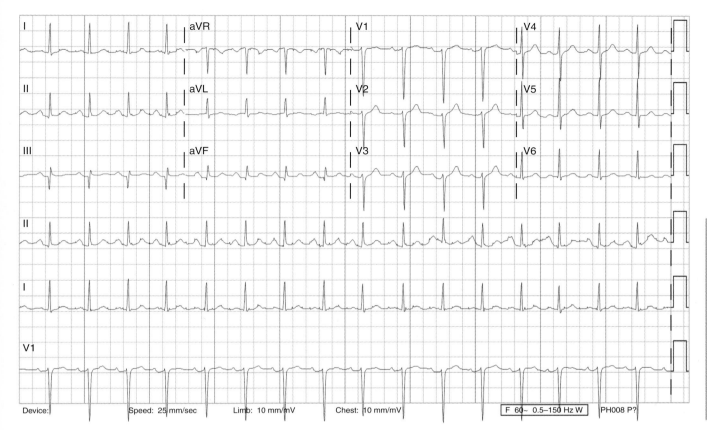

Device: Speed: 25 mm/sec   Limb: 10 mm/mV   Chest: 10 mm/mV   F 60~ 0.5–150 Hz W   PH008 P?

1. A 30-year-old woman presents to her primary care physician with complaints of occasional palpitations occurring over the last 10 years. She currently is asymptomatic and has no significant past medical, family, or social history. The electrocardiogram (ECG) shows:

A. Atrial tachycardia with inferior infarct, age indeterminate
B. Atrial tachycardia
C. Atrioventricular reentrant tachycardia
D. Sinus tachycardia with inferior infarct, age indeterminate
E. Sinus tachycardia with borderline poor R wave progression

 Notes

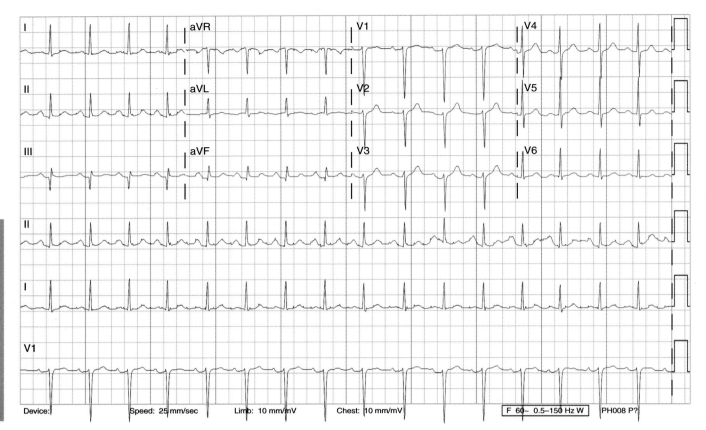

Device: Speed: 25 mm/sec   Limb: 10 mm/mV   Chest: 10 mm/mV   F 60~ 0.5–150 Hz W   PH008 P?

1. **The answer is E: Sinus tachycardia with borderline poor R wave progression.** Poor R wave progression is defined as the absence of transition from a negative to positive QRS complex in the precordial leads by lead V4. Borderline poor R wave progression can be defined as transition appropriately occurring by lead V4, but inappropriately delayed positive voltage transition from V1 to V3, as in this case. Poor R wave progression can be found in patients with anterior myocardial infarction, left ventricular hypertrophy, and in normal individuals. Sometimes it occurs due to lead misplacement, which is most likely the case in this patient given the clinical history. In fact, this patient's echocardiogram revealed normal wall motion and overall function.

A, B. This is not atrial tachycardia, because the P waves have an axis consistent with a sinus node origin in the high right atrium (positive P waves in lead II). Rarely an atrial tachycardia could be coming from near the sinus node and be indistinguishable from sinus tachycardia. In this situation, seeing the onset or offset of the tachycardia would distinguish sinus tachycardia from atrial tachycardia—sinus tachycardia begins and ends slowly, whereas atrial tachycardia begins and ends suddenly. **C.** When there are narrow QRS complexes, atrioventricular reentrant tachycardia (AVRT) would have retrograde (inverted in lead II) P waves with a different axis. AVRT involves conduction through an accessory bypass tract as part of the reentry circuit. **D.** This ECG is not consistent with an inferior infarct. Pathologic Q waves are defined as having a duration greater than 30 ms (~1 small box) and deeper than 0.1 mV (>1 small box) in two contiguous leads. Though the Q wave in lead III meets part of the criteria, the small Q wave in lead aVF does not. Many patients will have an isolated Q wave in lead III, and this is not pathologic.

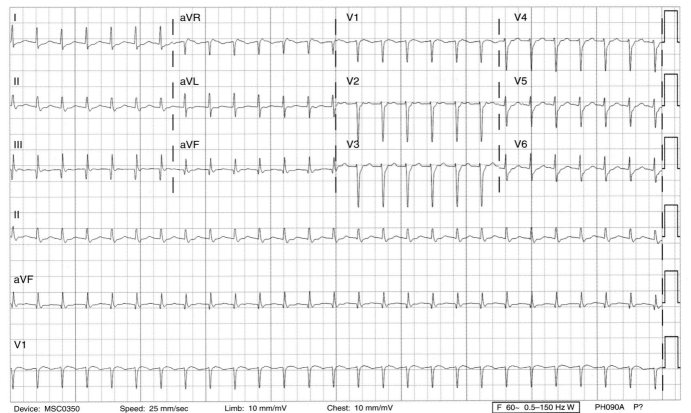

Device: MSC0350   Speed: 25 mm/sec   Limb: 10 mm/mV   Chest: 10 mm/mV   F 60~ 0.5–150 Hz W   PH090A   P?

2. The same 30-year-old woman presents to the emergency department 1 month later with the sudden onset of palpitations and mild lightheadedness. She had experienced briefer episodes over the last 10 years, but this episode persisted for 5 minutes. There has been no interval change in her nonsignificant past medical, family, or social history. Her physical exam is normal except for tachycardia. The ECG shows:

A. Sinus tachycardia
B. Ventricular tachycardia (VT)
C. Atrial flutter
D. Atrioventricular nodal reentrant tachycardia (AVNRT)
E. Wolff-Parkinson-White syndrome

✎ *Notes*

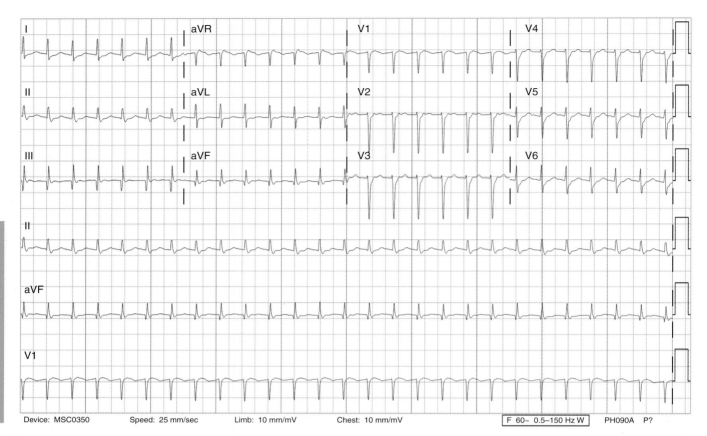

Device: MSC0350   Speed: 25 mm/sec   Limb: 10 mm/mV   Chest: 10 mm/mV | F 60~ 0.5–150 Hz W | PH090A   P?

2. **The answer is D: Atrioventricular nodal reentrant tachycardia (AVNRT).** This ECG shows AVNRT (also known as *atrioventricular nodal reciprocating tachycardia*), and poor R wave progression. The Q waves in leads III and aVF are not present in lead II and therefore do not reflect an infarct pattern. AVNRT is a supraventricular tachycardia that commonly occurs in adults with no structural heart disease, most commonly females in the third to fourth decade of life. It presents with palpitations and dizziness, sometimes with dyspnea and chest pain, and rarely syncope. Rates are typically between 140-250 bpm. AVNRT is a reentrant arrhythmia involving the AV node and perinodal tissue with anterograde conduction in a slow pathway and retrograde up a fast pathway, causing near-simultaneous activation of the atria and ventricles. As a result, there may be a inverted P wave noted, most commonly immediately following the QRS complex in the form of a pseudo-S wave, as seen in this tracing in the inferior and left precordial leads (though in some cases this P wave will be buried in the QRS complex or, less commonly,

immediately before the QRS). It is helpful to have a baseline ECG for comparison, at which point the retrograde P waves become clearly evident (see question 1, which depicts this patient's baseline ECG which lacks the retrograde P waves).

A. This ECG is not sinus tachycardia because of the lack of upright P waves in lead II preceding the QRS complex.
B. The QRS complexes are narrow and therefore not VT.
C. The rate of about 150 should prompt the thought of atrial flutter with 2:1 conduction, but there are no flutter waves present.
E. Wolff-Parkinson-White syndrome is the combination of preexcitation (exhibited by a short PR interval and a delta wave due to the faster conduction over the accessory pathway fusing with normal conduction through the AV node), and arrhythmias such as paroxysmal atrioventricular reentrant tachycardia (also known as *atrioventricular reciprocating tachycardia*). This case lacks a delta wave on the baseline ECG seen in question 1.

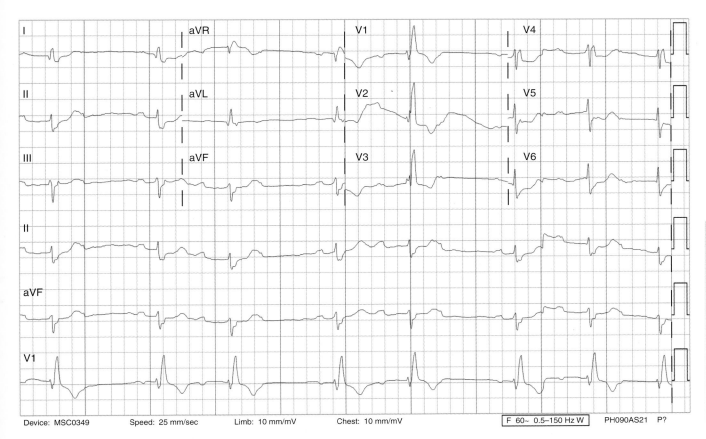

Device: MSC0349   Speed: 25 mm/sec   Limb: 10 mm/mV   Chest: 10 mm/mV   F 60~ 0.5–150 Hz W   PH090AS21   P?

3. A 63-year-old man presents to your office with complaints of intermittent lightheadedness without syncope. He has type 2 diabetic, is hypertensive, and has gout but has no known cardiac disease. His ECG shows:

Notes

A. Sinus rhythm, first-degree AV block, intermittent blocked atrial premature complexes, right bundle branch block, and left anterior fascicular block

B. Sinus rhythm, Mobitz type I second-degree AV block, right bundle branch block, and left anterior fascicular block

C. Sinus rhythm, Mobitz type II second-degree AV block, right bundle branch block, and left posterior fascicular block

D. Sinus rhythm, third-degree AV block, ventricular escape rhythm

E. Accelerated idioventricular rhythm with AV dissociation

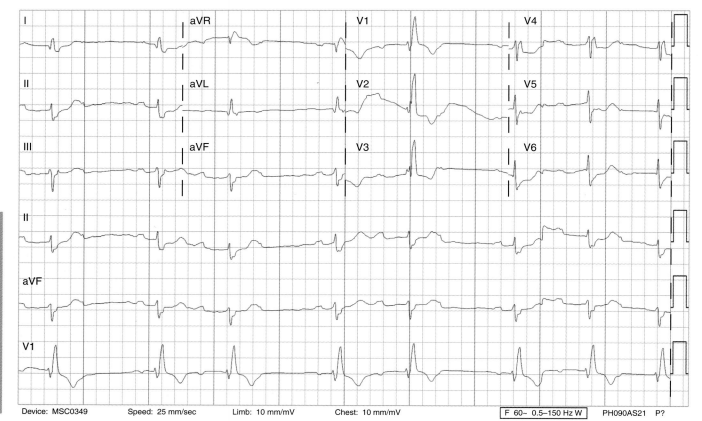

Device: MSC0349   Speed: 25 mm/sec   Limb: 10 mm/mV   Chest: 10 mm/mV   F 60~ 0.5–150 Hz W   PH090AS21 P?

3. **The answer is B: Sinus rhythm, Mobitz type I second-degree AV block, right bundle branch block, and left anterior fascicular block.** This is bradycardia with an atrial rate just above 60 bpm, with lengthening of the PR interval before dropping QRS complexes. Note there are P waves seen at the end of the T waves of the 3rd, 5th and 7th beats (seen best in rhythm lead aVF), with no conduction after the 3rd and 5th beats, and even longer PR prolongation after the 7th beat, all consistent with Mobitz type I second-degree AV block. The QRS duration >120 ms (>3 small boxes), the rSR′ in lead V1, and the deep, wide S waves in lead V6 and lead I are all consistent with right bundle branch block. Left axis deviation in the absence of left ventricular hypertrophy, inferior infarct, or left bundle branch block is consistent with left anterior fascicular block. There is also left atrial enlargement defined by a P wave >120 ms (>3 small boxes) and/or two positive deflections separated by >40 ms (>1 small box) in lead II, and/or a P wave with a negative deflection in lead V1 that is >40 ms (>1 small box) and deeper than 0.1 mV (>1 small box).

Mobitz type I second-degree AV block occurs within the AV node and is commonly asymptomatic, not requiring treatment. This patient was symptomatic with evidence of other conduction system disease (right bundle branch block and left anterior fascicular block) and therefore requires a pacemaker.

A. This is not first-degree AV block with blocked atrial premature contractions because none of the P waves are premature (they are regular), and the pattern of progressive PR lengthening before the dropped QRS complex is consistent with Mobitz type I second-degree AV block.
C. Mobitz type II second-degree AV block lacks progressive PR lengthening manifesting as random, unpredictable drops of QRS complexes. This degree of heart block is considered higher grade (below the AV node) and often will necessitate a pacemaker. Left posterior fascicular block, not present here, is defined as right axis deviation greater than 100 degrees in the absence of right ventricular hypertrophy, pulmonary embolism, lateral wall infarct, dextrocardia, or lead reversal.
D. Third-degree AV block requires complete AV dissociation, with the atrial rate going faster than the ventricular rate. Ventricular escape rates are usually less than 40 bpm and are fairly regular.
E. Accelerated idioventricular arrhythmia is classically seen as an asymptomatic ventricular tachyarrhythmia following the opening of an acutely occluded coronary artery with thrombolytics or percutaneous coronary intervention. They are faster than a ventricular escape rhythm, but slower than VT and ordinarily resolve on their own without treatment.

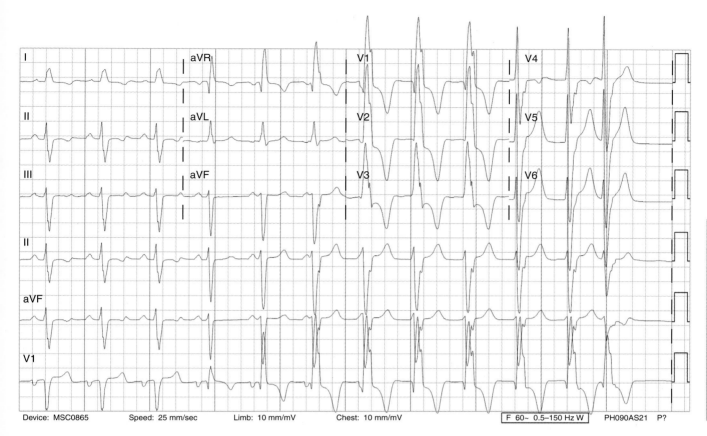

Device: MSC0865   Speed: 25 mm/sec   Limb: 10 mm/mV   Chest: 10 mm/mV   F 60~ 0.5–150 Hz W   PH090AS21   P?

4. A 58-year-old man with a history of medically managed coronary artery disease, end-stage renal disease, hypertension, and diabetes presented with 2 weeks of intermittent shortness of breath with exertion. On the day of admission, he developed substernal chest discomfort described as, "Someone stepping on me." In the emergency department, he was found to have a new left bundle branch block and went urgently to the catheterization lab where he was found to have a completely occluded proximal left anterior descending artery that was opened successfully with a bare metal stent. Thirty minutes after his intervention, the patient has this ECG done in the coronary care unit. What is the most reasonable next step?

A. Continue observation
B. Start intravenous (IV) amiodarone
C. Prepare the patient urgently for cardioversion
D. Call the interventional cardiologist to transport emergently back to the catheterization lab for repeat angioplasty
E. Have transcutaneous pacing pads placed on the patient, and the pacemaker on stand-by

 Notes

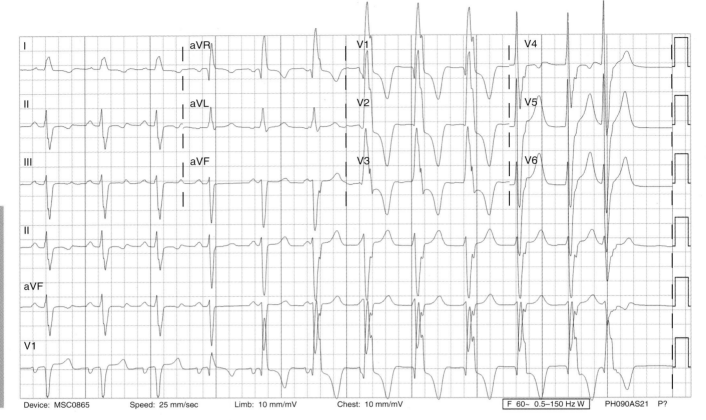

| Device: MSC0865 | Speed: 25 mm/sec | Limb: 10 mm/mV | Chest: 10 mm/mV | F 60~ 0.5–150 Hz W | PH090AS21 P? |

4. **The answer is A: Continue observation.** This ECG reveals sinus rhythm, left atrial enlargement, first-degree AV block, left bundle branch block, prolonged QT, with the onset of an accelerated idioventricular rhythm (AIVR) starting with the fourth beat, and a ventricular premature complex (the last beat). Note there is AV dissociation, an indication of a ventricular source of arrhythmia, as the sinus P waves march through the rhythm strip at the bottom. By the 6th beat, the P wave is not responsible for the ventricular complex (the PR interval is too short), and by the 11th beat, you can see the P wave as a small negative deflection at the end of the QRS complex (see lead V1). The last recorded beat comes in early, but appears to be coming from the same focus as the AIVR. Note that it is followed immediately by what appears to be a retrograde P wave tucked in on the end of the QRS complex (best seen as a positive deflection in rhythm lead V1, and a negative deflection in rhythm leads II and aVF). There is then a compensatory pause with lack of regular sinus activity (blocked by the retrograde P wave). In AIVR, the ventricular rate is often between 60 and 110 bpm, frequently within 10 beats of the sinus rhythm with shift between the two occurring frequently as they compete for dominance. Fusion beats (4th and 5th beats) are QRS complexes with morphology between the ventricular beats and the normally conducted sinus beats as impulses from both fuse to form the complex, another marker indicating a ventricular source for the arrhythmia. AIVR is most often seen after an acutely occluded coronary artery is opened with thrombolytics or balloon angioplasty with or without stenting and is due to enhanced automaticity. It ordinarily requires no treatment and subsides on its own. Lastly AIVR can also be seen in digitalis toxicity, which can be treated with digoxin immune Fab (immunoglobulin fragments) acutely.

B, C, D, E. Ordinarily the patient is asymptomatic and requires no further treatment.

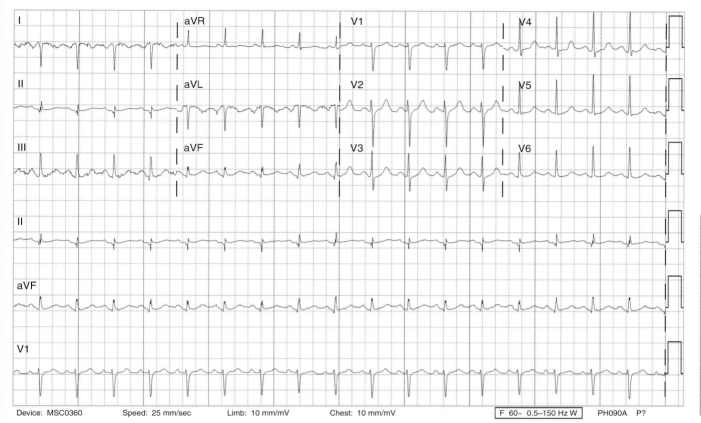

Device: MSC0360   Speed: 25 mm/sec   Limb: 10 mm/mV   Chest: 10 mm/mV   F 60~ 0.5–150 Hz W   PH090A   P?

5. You are asked to see a 52-year-old woman with no prior medical history admitted to the neurosurgery service with a nontraumatic subarachnoid bleed. She was just placed on a ventilator, and an urgent craniotomy is planned. Based on the above ECG done 2 hours earlier, what would be the next best step before proceeding to surgery?

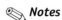 *Notes*

A. Echocardiogram to assess for right ventricular hypokinesis
B. Repeat ECG
C. Look at the chest x-ray to confirm a congenital heart abnormality
D. Stress test to assess for significant ischemia
E. β-blocker

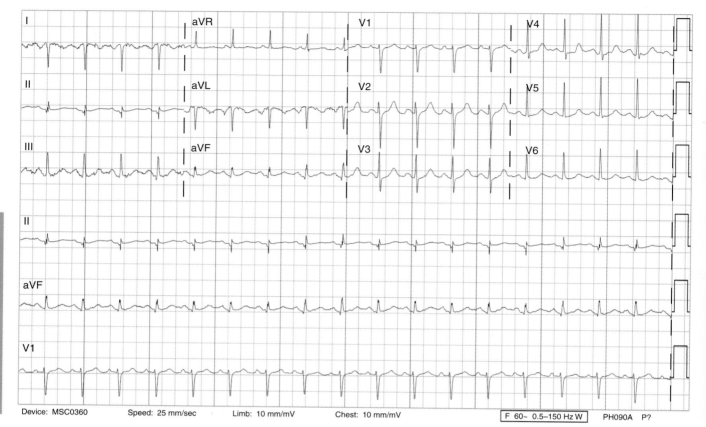

Device: MSC0360   Speed: 25 mm/sec   Limb: 10 mm/mV   Chest: 10 mm/mV   F 60~ 0.5–150 Hz W   PH090A P?

5. **The answer is B: Repeat ECG.** This ECG demonstrates sinus tachycardia with apparent right axis deviation. However, make note that the predominantly positive precordial P waves appear to support a sinus mechanism from the high right atrium, but the negative P waves in I and flat P waves in II do not. This suggests limb lead reversal. With right arm–left arm lead reversal, as in this case, lead I is inverted, leads II and III are reversed, leads aVR and aVL are reversed, and lead aVF is unchanged. Right arm left–arm lead reversal is one of the more common reasons for right axis deviation, and assessing the P wave morphology as explained helps distinguish this. This abnormality needs to be distinguished from rare dextrocardia, which can also produce these limb lead findings. However, the precordial leads would show lack of normal R wave progression as the heart would be in the other side of the chest.

A. Despite what appears to be right axis deviation at first, there is no evidence of right ventricular hypertrophy or enlargement on this ECG, and therefore echocardiogram is not indicated.
C. As the ECG pattern is most consistent with limb lead reversal, the chest x-ray is unlikely to be helpful, unless there was lack of precordial R wave transition in which dextrocardia would be more likely.
D. There is no role for a stress test in this patient who has an urgent noncardiac surgical indication.
E. There are no findings to suggest that β-blocker therapy is indicated.

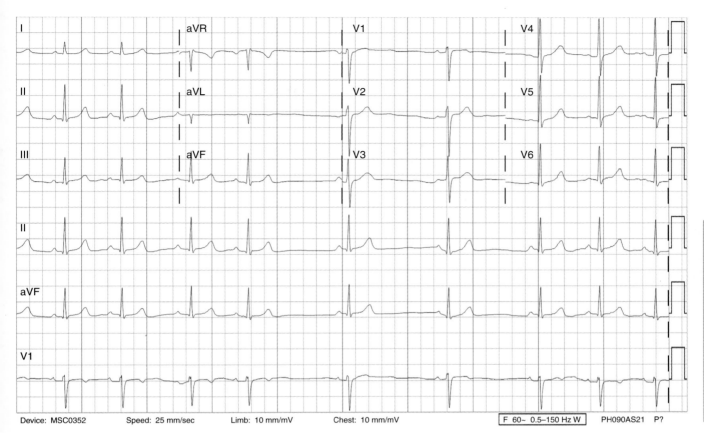

Device: MSC0352   Speed: 25 mm/sec   Limb: 10 mm/mV   Chest: 10 mm/mV   F 60~ 0.5–150 Hz W   PH090AS21 P?

6. A 24-year-old female heroin abuser presents with fever and malaise. She has been complaining of mild palpitations. She is normotensive, has a normal pulse oximetry on room air, but has a holosystolic murmur heard at the right lower sternal border. An ECG is performed. What would be the best next step?

 Notes

A. Repeat ECG now
B. Echocardiogram
C. Give 1 mg of IV atropine
D. Have transcutaneous pacing pads placed on the patient, and the pacemaker on standby
E. CT scan of the chest

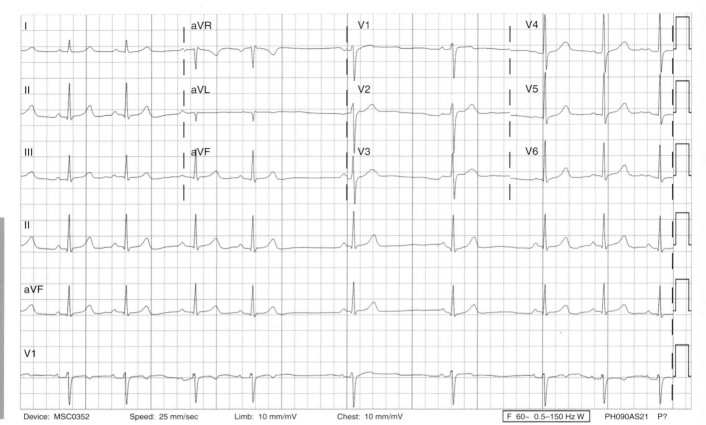

Device: MSC0352   Speed: 25 mm/sec   Limb: 10 mm/mV   Chest: 10 mm/mV   F 60~ 0.5–150 Hz W   PH090AS21 P?

6. **The answer is B: Echocardiogram.** This patient's ECG demonstrates sinus arrhythmia, which commonly occurs in the younger patient, and is due to normal, enhanced vagal tone. The P-P interval shortens during inspiration, due to reflex inhibition of vagal tone, and lengthens during expiration. Very rarely, sinus arrhythmia is symptomatic if the P-P interval is excessively long. Following blood cultures and antibiotic initiation, a transthoracic echocardiogram is the most reasonable next step given the IV drug abuse history, the fever, and the murmur suggestive of tricuspid valve regurgitation.

A. There is no reason to immediately repeat an ECG. Daily ECGs, however, are reasonable if there is concern or confirmation of aortic valve vegetations, as these could progress to aortic valve abscess and AV nodal block, often first manifest as first-degree AV block.
C, D, E. There is no immediate indication for atropine, transcutaneous pacing, or CT scan.

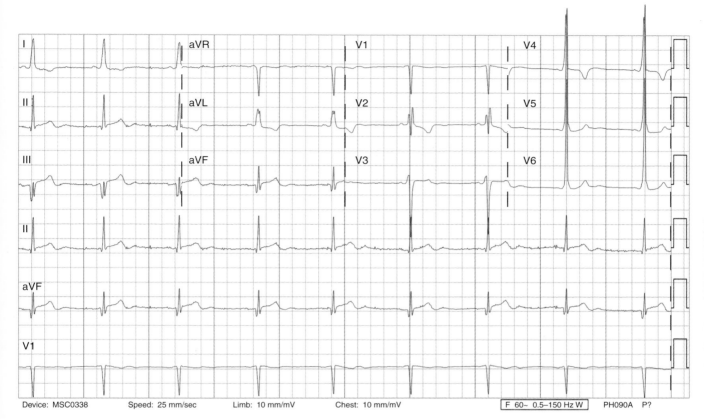

Device: MSC0338   Speed: 25 mm/sec   Limb: 10 mm/mV   Chest: 10 mm/mV   F 60~ 0.5–150 Hz W   PH090A   P?

7. A 23-year-old man with no past medical history presents to the emergency department with syncope. He has a normal physical exam. Based on the ECG, the most appropriate next step would be:

A. Placement of a transvenous pacemaker
B. Referral for coronary angiography and angioplasty if indicated
C. Initiation of IV amiodarone
D. Referral for neurologic evaluation and electroencephalography (EEG)
E. Referral for electrophysiology study

 Notes

Section II CARDIOLOGY

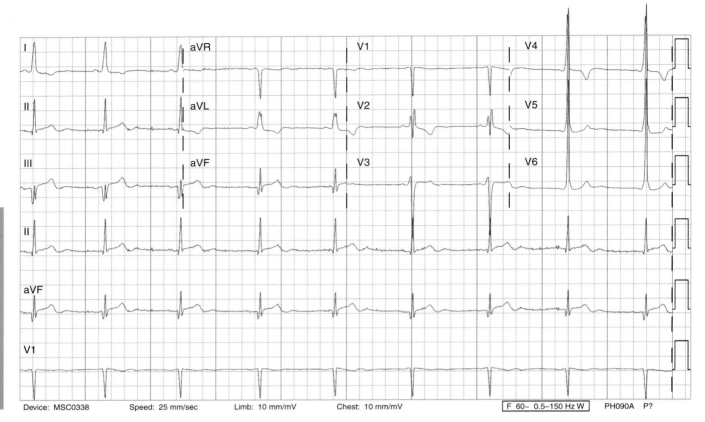

Device: MSC0338   Speed: 25 mm/sec   Limb: 10 mm/mV   Chest: 10 mm/mV   F 60~ 0.5–150 Hz W   PH090A   P?

7. **The answer is E: Referral for electrophysiology study.**
This ECG shows sinus bradycardia, a delta wave
consistent with preexcitation from a bypass tract
(short PR interval, slurring of the initial QRS), and a
pseudoinfarct pattern inferoposteriorly (Q waves and
ST elevation in II/aVF). The presence of a preexcitation
pattern with documented arrhythmias such as AVRT
is known as Wolf-Parkinson-White syndrome. Given
this ECG pattern and a history of syncope, there is high
concern for more lethal arrhythmias that involve the
bypass tract, such as atrial fibrillation that could conduct
so quickly down the bypass tract to the ventricles as to
cause VT, ventricular fibrillation, and sudden death.
An electrophysiology study is indicated with possible
radiofrequency ablation of the bypass tract.

A. There is no indication for transvenous pacemaker
based on this ECG.
B. Coronary angiography is not indicated. The
Q waves seen inferiorly with evidence of posterior
involvement (prominent early R wave in V2) are, in
fact, preexcitation delta waves indicative of the bypass
tract (pseudoinfarct pattern).
C. Amiodarone would be a good choice if there was
evidence of rapid atrial fibrillation or AVRT, neither of
which have been documented yet in this patient.
D. Neurologic evaluation with EEG is certainly a
reasonable step in many patients with syncope.
However, with this ECG pattern, cardiac syncope is
more likely.

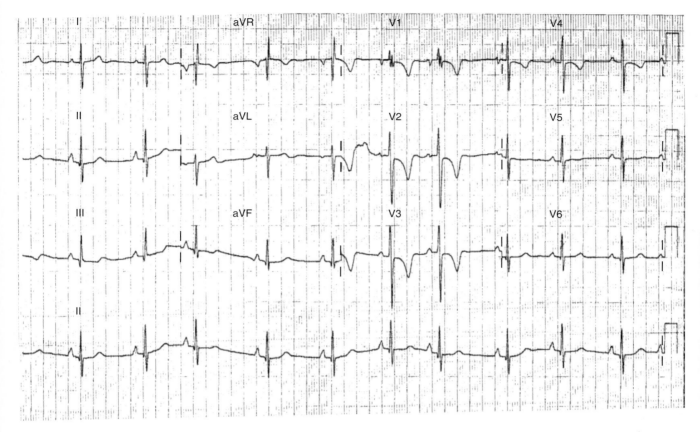

8. A 25-year-old man complains of 2 years of mildly progressive dyspnea on exertion. He presents for further evaluation, mostly at the insistence of his fiancée. His exam is notable for a prominent S2 heart sound and a systolic ejection murmur at the left upper sternal border with a subtle heave noted on palpation of the precordium. His ECG shows:

A. Sinus arrhythmia, right axis deviation, right atrial enlargement, right ventricular hypertrophy with strain pattern

B. Sinus rhythm with premature atrial complexes, left axis deviation, left atrial enlargement, right bundle branch block

C. Sinus arrhythmia, left axis deviation, left atrial enlargement, left ventricular hypertrophy with strain pattern

D. Wandering atrial pacemaker, right bundle branch block

E. Sinus rhythm, left axis deviation, ischemic T wave abnormalities

✎ *Notes*

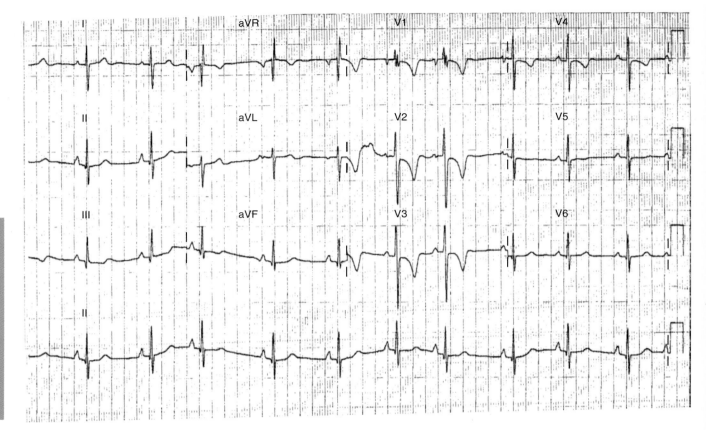

8. **The answer is A: Sinus arrhythmia, right axis deviation, right atrial enlargement, right ventricular hypertrophy with strain pattern.** This pattern is consistent with right ventricular hypertrophy. There is right axis deviation defined as a QRS axis >100 degrees: note the S wave is deeper than the height of the R wave in lead I with predominantly positive QRS complexes in the inferior leads. Right atrial enlargement is defined as a tall P wave >0.25 mV (>2.5 small boxes) in lead II (seen here), and/or a tall P wave in lead V1 >0.15 mV (>1.5 small boxes). Right ventricular hypertrophy is seen with a prominent R wave that is taller than the small S wave in lead V1, relatively deep S waves in leads V5 and V6, a tall dominant R wave in lead aVR, with deep T wave inversions in leads V1 to V4 consistent with a strain pattern. On echocardiogram, this patient was found to have an enlarged right atrium, a hypertrophied and dilated right ventricle, and a pulmonary artery systolic pressure of 80 mm Hg. He was diagnosed with *cor*

pulmonale secondary to idiopathic pulmonary arterial hypertension.

B, C, D, E. The rhythm is irregular due to sinus arrhythmia, not premature atrial contractions or wandering atrial pacemaker. The axis is not leftward given the predominantly negative deflection in lead I. Sometimes *cor pulmonale* can be associated with an incomplete or complete right bundle branch block. However, as in the ECG above, there is no true rSR', and the QRS is narrow, excluding right bundle branch block. The notching of the downslope of the R wave in lead V1 is consistent with a delayed intrinsicoid (delayed time of the downslope after the R wave) which is also seen in right ventricular hypertrophy. Though the P wave in lead V1 appears to be deeper than 0.1 mV (>1 small box) it is not quite as wide as 40 ms (>1 small box), making this borderline left atrial enlargement. The precordial T wave abnormalities are more consistent with a right ventricular strain pattern from the right ventricular hypertrophy in this ECG rather than ischemia.

ECG A

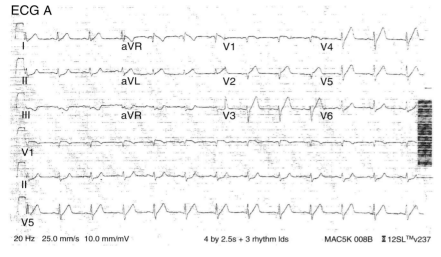

20 Hz   25.0 mm/s   10.0 mm/mV   4 by 2.5s + 3 rhythm lds   MAC5K 008B   ⚡12SL™v237

ECG B

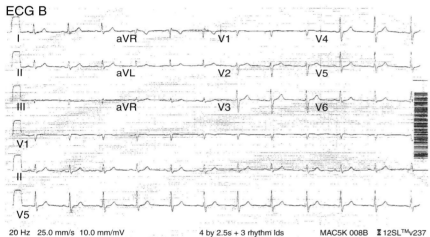

20 Hz   25.0 mm/s   10.0 mm/mV   4 by 2.5s + 3 rhythm lds   MAC5K 008B   ⚡12SL™v237

9. A 60-year-old man with hyperlipidemia taking over-the-counter fish oil supplements, and with a family history of a younger brother who had coronary artery bypass surgery, presented to an emergency department after experiencing jaw pain and upper chest tightness that started at the end of a routine 20-mile bike ride. ECG A was done at presentation (with chest pain), while ECG B was done 5 minutes later after sublingual nitroglycerin resolved the pain. Based on these ECGs, the most likely diagnosis is:

A. High grade left anterior descending artery stenosis
B. High grade right coronary artery stenosis
C. Hyperkalemia
D. Hyperventilation
E. Acute pulmonary embolus

 Notes

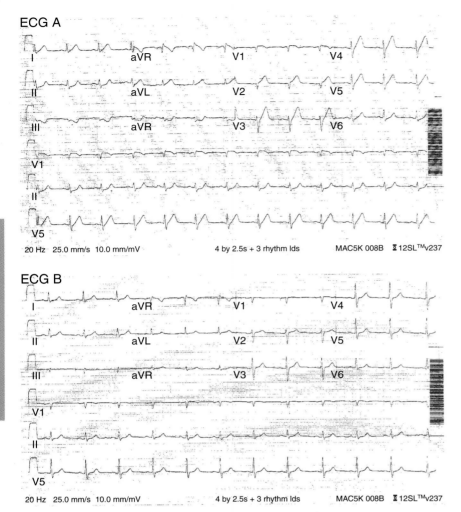

ECG A

I aVR V1 V4
II aVL V2 V5
III aVR V3 V6
V1
II
V5

20 Hz 25.0 mm/s 10.0 mm/mV 4 by 2.5s + 3 rhythm lds MAC5K 008B ⊠ 12SL™v237

ECG B

I aVR V1 V4
II aVL V2 V5
III aVR V3 V6
V1
II
V5

20 Hz 25.0 mm/s 10.0 mm/mV 4 by 2.5s + 3 rhythm lds MAC5K 008B ⊠ 12SL™v237

9. **The answer is A: High grade left anterior descending artery stenosis.** ECG A shows sinus rhythm with broad based prominent T waves in the precordial leads (called *hyperacute T waves*), inferior lead ST segment depression, and ST segment elevation in lead aVR, all consistent with diffuse subendocardial ischemia, likely from a high grade left anterior descending artery stenosis. Comparing ECG A to a prior ECG, or in this case, an ECG done 5 minutes later (ECG B) once chest pain resolved is important in identifying these dynamic ECG changes. ECG B shows resolution of the T wave and ST segment changes. The patient went on to the catheterization lab and a 70% mid-left anterior descending artery stenosis with associated thrombus was successfully stented. His precatheterization troponin was mildly elevated, and he did have mid- to distal-anteroseptal, anterior, and apical akinesis on echocardiogram due to myocardial stunning during ischemia. When ischemia is likely by clinical history and hyperacute, negative, or biphasic T waves are present in the precordial leads, this suggests high grade left anterior descending artery stenosis and should be treated aggressively.

B. Though there are ST segment depressions in the inferior leads, the depression does not correlate with territory of ischemia as the ST segment elevation does. These represent reciprocal changes: ST depression in inferior leads during anteroseptal ischemia or ST depression in the anterior leads during inferoposterior ischemia. Hyperacute precordial T waves are not typically seen with right coronary artery stenoses.
C. The more broad based, rounded T waves (hyperacute T waves) here are not consistent with hyperkalemia, which usually would have sharp symmetrically peaked T waves, shortening of the QT interval, and sometimes ST segment elevation.
D, E. Hyperventilation and acute pulmonary embolus can cause ST segment and T wave changes, but not typically hyperacute T waves.

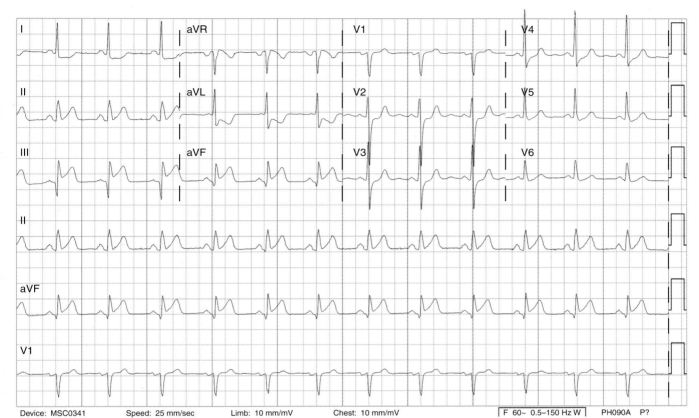

I	aVR	V1	V4
II	aVL	V2	V5
III	aVF	V3	V6

II

aVF

V1

Device: MSC0341   Speed: 25 mm/sec   Limb: 10 mm/mV   Chest: 10 mm/mV   F 60~ 0.5–150 Hz W   PH090A   P?

10. You are called to see your patient in the emergency department. He is a 54-year-old man with a history of abnormal calcium score on a prior cardiac CT, hypertension on treatment, and a family history of premature coronary artery disease in his younger brother. He presents with severe chest pain and upper back pain described as a "clamp" that began 30 minutes earlier. His blood pressure is 198/96 mm Hg in the right arm, and 170/76 mm Hg in the left arm. His exam is otherwise unremarkable except for diaphoresis and anxiety. An ECG is performed. Which would be the most appropriate next immediate step?

A. V/Q scan
B. IV thrombolytic therapy
C. Start IV heparin now, followed by IV eptifibatide if his troponin is elevated
D. A chest x-ray
E. IV nifedipine

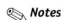 **Notes**

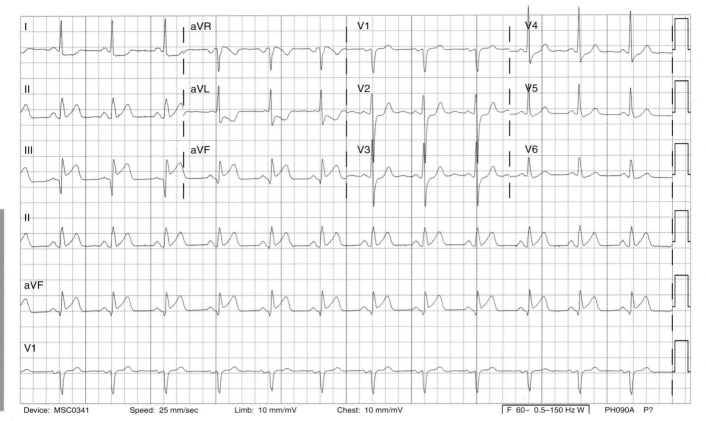

Device: MSC0341   Speed: 25 mm/sec   Limb: 10 mm/mV   Chest: 10 mm/mV   F 60~ 0.5–150 Hz W   PH090A   P?

10. **The answer is D: A chest x-ray.** This ECG reveals sinus rhythm with ST elevation consistent with an acute inferior injury pattern and reciprocal lateral ST depression. In the vast majority of cases, there should be no delay in opening the occluded vessel with either IV thrombolytics (under 30 minutes from presentation) or coronary angioplasty and stent (under 90 minutes). Before proceeding emergently, however, it is always imperative to exclude any contraindications. In this patient with chest and back pain and a more than 20 mm Hg difference in arm blood pressures, ascending aortic dissection needs to be rapidly excluded. If a widened mediastinum is noted on chest x-ray, then emergent confirmatory imaging with either CT angiography of the aorta or transesophageal echocardiography could be done while cardiothoracic surgery is emergently consulted for a life-threatening aortic dissection. Alternatively, an aortogram could be performed at the beginning of a cardiac catheterization. If the mediastinum was not widened on chest x-ray, but the clinical suspicion remains high, further diagnostic studies should be rapidly performed before giving thrombolytics,

anticoagulation, or IV antiplatelet agents. In this case, an aortic dissection was confirmed on CT angiogram, and the patient was transported to a hospital with a cardiothoracic surgeon. Ascending aortic dissection carries a mortality rate that increases approximately 2% per hour after presentation. Aortic dissections can sometimes present with an acute injury pattern such as this if the dissection flap occludes flow into the right coronary artery (which occurs more commonly than into the left).

A. There is no role for a V/Q scan to look for pulmonary embolus in this scenario.
B, C. IV thrombolytics are absolutely contraindicated in suspected aortic dissection, and IV heparin could worsen the dissection acutely.
E. IV nifedipine would not be a good choice as this could actually cause a reflex increase in cardiac contractility, possibly worsening the extent of an aortic dissection. A continuous IV β-blocker would be the first agent of choice to rapidly control the blood pressure while diagnostic tests are performed.

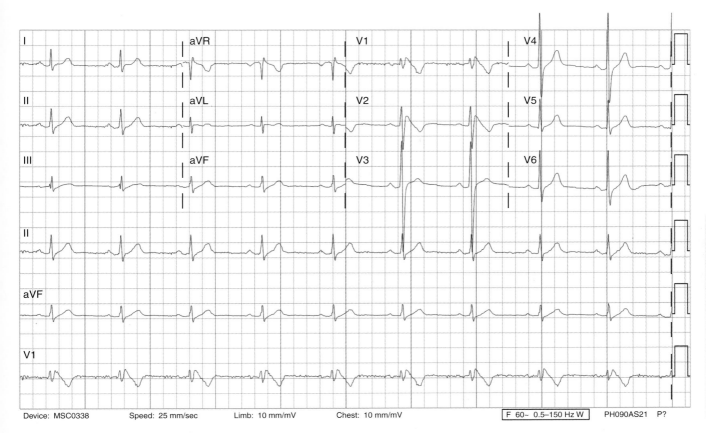

Device: MSC0338   Speed: 25 mm/sec   Limb: 10 mm/mV   Chest: 10 mm/mV   F 60~ 0.5–150 Hz W   PH090AS21   P?

11. A 37-year-old male with a history of seizures since age 15 and migraines, presents to your office with complaints of palpitations that awoke him from sleep the night before and associated near-syncope. This occurred off and on over a few hours. He has had similar symptoms sporadically in the past several years, but this episode was more intense. He describes them as different from his seizures. His exam is normal. Based on the ECG above, the most appropriate recommendation is:

A. 24-hour outpatient continuous ECG monitoring
B. Electrophysiology study
C. Follow-up with his neurologist
D. Stress test
E. Admission to the hospital for emergent coronary angiography and angioplasty if indicated

 Notes

Section II CARDIOLOGY

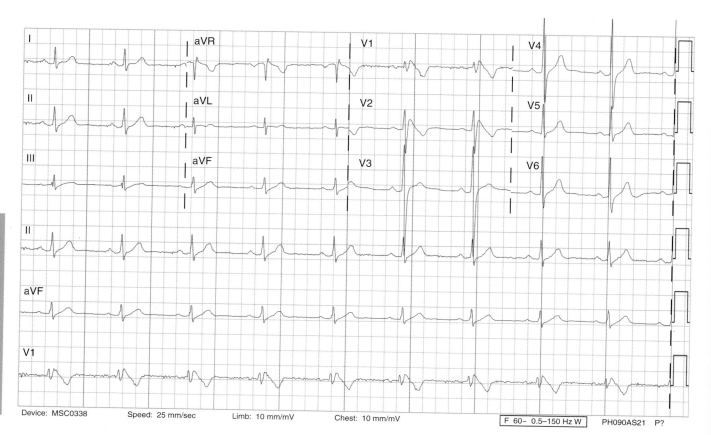

Device: MSC0338   Speed: 25 mm/sec   Limb: 10 mm/mV   Chest: 10 mm/mV   F 60~ 0.5–150 Hz W   PH090AS21   P?

11. **The answer is B: Electrophysiology study.** An electrophysiology study is indicated in this particular patient with near-syncope because the ECG shows sinus rhythm with ST elevation in leads V1 and V2 consistent with a Brugada pattern. Brugada syndrome with this ECG pattern is associated with ventricular arrhythmias and sudden arrhythmic death. Classically it is characterized by a prominent coved ST elevation greater than 0.2 mV (>2 small boxes) ending with a negative T wave in leads V1 and V2. Alternatively, and more subtly, this ST elevation more than 0.2 mV (>2 small boxes) can then sag in the middle of the ST segment >0.1 mV or <0.1 mV (> or <1 small box) above baseline, ending with a positive or biphasic T wave (termed *saddle-back variations*). The prevalence in the United States is not well established, but in Asia this syndrome is the most likely cause of sudden

death in men younger than 50 years of age. It is at least eight times more prevalent in men than in women. Syncope and sudden death are common. The family history is important, though the syndrome can occur sporadically. It is due to a mutation in the *SCN5A* gene that encodes for a voltage-gated sodium channel. Treatment is an implantable cardioverter-defibrillator to prevent sudden death.

A, C. Given the presyncope with this concerning ECG pattern, electrophysiology study is warranted before 24-hour continuous ECG monitoring or neurology follow-up.

D, E. There is no indication for a stress test or coronary angiography, as the history and ST abnormalities are not typical of ischemia.

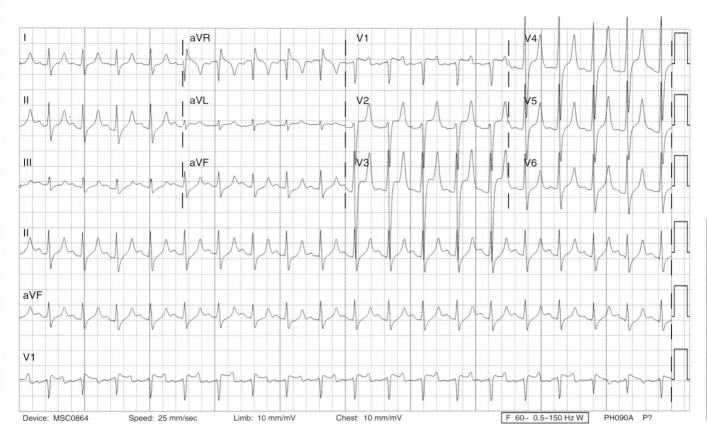

| Device: MSC0864 | Speed: 25 mm/sec | Limb: 10 mm/mV | Chest: 10 mm/mV | F 60~ 0.5–150 Hz W | PH090A   P? |

12. A 49-year-old patient with a history of sickle cell disease and cocaine abuse was admitted with intestinal ischemia and underwent urgent exploratory laparotomy and resection of the terminal ileum. Two days postoperatively, an ECG is performed. What would be the most appropriate next best step?

 Notes

A. Urgent coronary angiography
B. IV calcium gluconate
C. IV magnesium sulfate
D. IV sodium phosphate
E. Pulmonary embolus protocol CT

Section II CARDIOLOGY

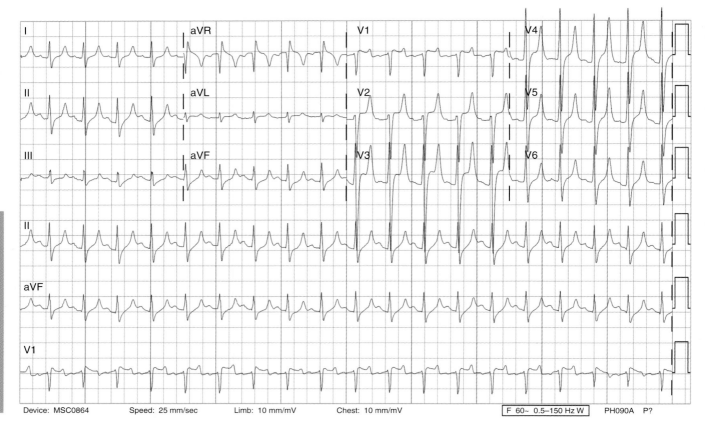

| Device: MSC0864 | Speed: 25 mm/sec | Limb: 10 mm/mV | Chest: 10 mm/mV | F 60~ 0.5–150 Hz W | PH090A | P? |

12. **The answer is B: IV calcium gluconate.** This ECG demonstrates sinus tachycardia, borderline intraventricular conduction delay, and peaked T waves consistent with hyperkalemia from lactic acidosis and renal failure. Calcium gluconate antagonizes the effects of potassium on myocardium, rapidly reducing the likelihood of arrhythmias, but it does not actually lower the potassium. Other measures such as insulin and dextrose infusions, sodium bicarbonate, and high-dose inhaled β-agonists will lower potassium by driving potassium from the extracellular space into cells. Sodium polystyrene sulfonate binds potassium in the intestinal tract but takes the longest to act. Lastly, in renal failure, hemodialysis is sometimes indicated if medical therapy fails. Hyperkalemia has a typical ECG progression. With potassium levels between 6 to 6.5 mEq/L, there are peaked T waves with a very pointy peak as in this example. From 6.5 to 7 mEq/L, there is PR prolongation with flattening then loss of P waves. Greater than 8 mEq/L, there is widening of the QRS progressing to a sine-wave morphology followed by ventricular fibrillation and asystole.

A, C, D, E. There is no role for coronary angiography, as the J-point elevation seen in leads V1 through V3 is likely due to the hyperkalemia. Additionally, the ST segment is not convex up as would be more typical of an acute injury pattern. IV magnesium sulfate, potassium phosphate, or a pulmonary embolus protocol CT are not indicated.

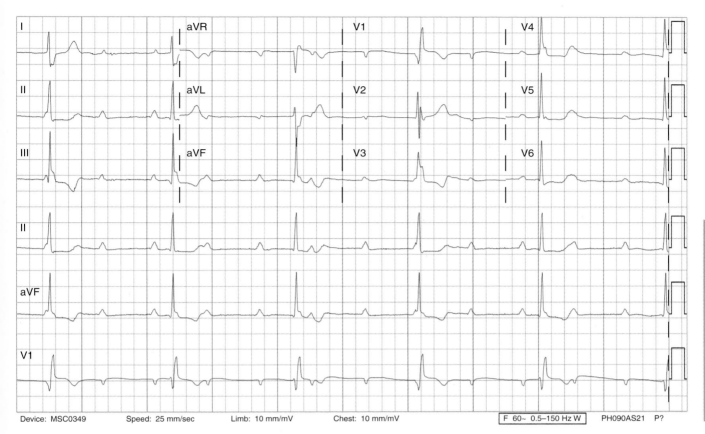

Device: MSC0349   Speed: 25 mm/sec   Limb: 10 mm/mV   Chest: 10 mm/mV   F 60~ 0.5–150 Hz W   PH090AS21   P?

13. A 47-year-old woman with hypertension treated with atenolol presents to your office complaining of fatigue and dyspnea with exertion that she notices on her morning hikes through the woods over the last week. She has no complaints at rest. On review of systems, she does report rashes in the past, but she could not recall if they were bull's eye–shaped. She does report frequently removing ticks from her dog. On exam, her pulse rate is slow, but there are no rashes. Based on her ECG, what would be the best recommendation?

 Notes

A. Decrease the atenolol dose and follow up in 1 week
B. Admission to the hospital for placement of a permanent pacemaker
C. Admission to the hospital for observation and possible placement of a transvenous pacemaker
D. Check Lyme titers with close outpatient follow-up
E. Admission to the hospital for urgent coronary angiogram with angioplasty if indicated

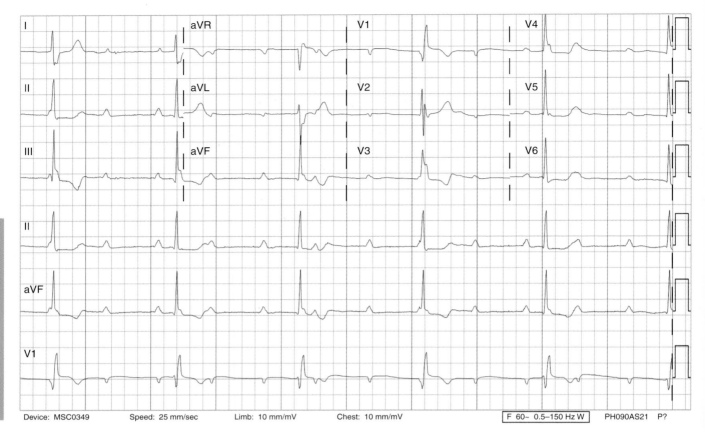

Device: MSC0349   Speed: 25 mm/sec   Limb: 10 mm/mV   Chest: 10 mm/mV   F 60~ 0.5–150 Hz W   PH090AS21   P?

13. **The answer is C: Admission to the hospital for observation and possible placement of a transvenous pacemaker.** The ECG shows sinus rhythm with left atrial enlargement, third-degree AV block, and a fascicular escape rhythm in the 30s. Given the high-grade AV block with an escape rhythm well below the AV node, she is at high risk for syncope and sudden death. Therefore admission to the hospital for consideration of a transvenous pacemaker is appropriate.

A. This is an unstable rhythm, and though stopping the atenolol is appropriate, allowing for outpatient follow-up is inappropriate.

B, D. Given her history, checking Lyme titers on admission to the hospital (not as an outpatient) would be reasonable, because if this is heart block related to Lyme disease, with antibiotic treatment she may not require a permanent pacemaker.
E. Although coronary artery disease and ischemia can lead to heart block, there is nothing in her history or ECG that warrants urgent coronary angiography.

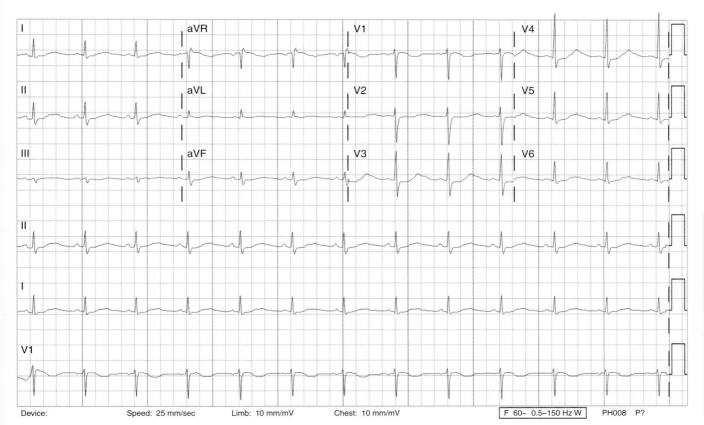

Device: Speed: 25 mm/sec   Limb: 10 mm/mV   Chest: 10 mm/mV   F 60~ 0.5–150 Hz W   PH008   P?

14. A 28-year-old man presents for a checkup after his 25-year-old brother died suddenly while diving in the Caribbean Islands. Your patient's history is notable for one syncopal episode 4 years earlier, which was sudden and brief, without associated trauma. He did not seek medical care and thought it was due to heat exhaustion. He takes no medications and has no significant medical or social history. His exam is normal. His ECG is shown above. Which of the following can be associated with this ECG finding?

A. Hypercalcemia
B. Hyperkalemia
C. IV lidocaine
D. Erythromycin
E. Metoprolol

✎ *Notes*

Section II CARDIOLOGY

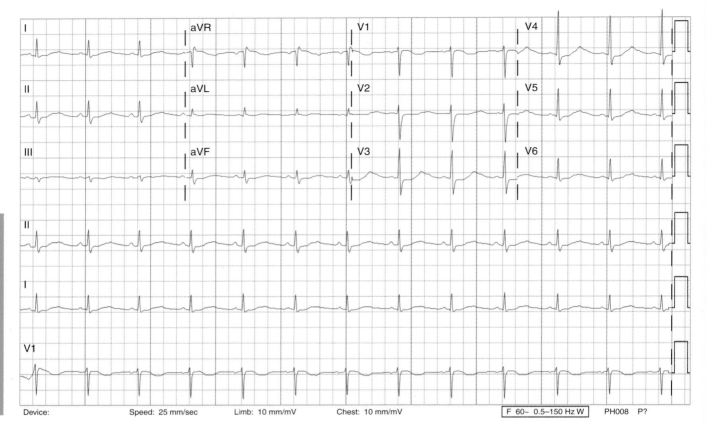

| Device: | Speed: 25 mm/sec | Limb: 10 mm/mV | Chest: 10 mm/mV | F 60~ 0.5–150 Hz W | PH008 P? |

14. **The answer is D: Erythromycin.** The ECG shows normal sinus rhythm with a markedly prolonged QT interval. QT prolongation is associated with polymorphic ventricular tachycardia (*torsades des pointes*) and death. Given the patient's age and family history of possible sudden cardiac death, congenital long QT syndrome is probable. There are other acquired causes of long QT, such as medications including erythromycin, clarithromycin, haloperidol, and methadone. For a complete list refer to *www.torsades.org*. In addition, other conditions may cause long QT such as ischemia, hypothyroidism, hypocalcemia, hypokalemia, and severe brain injury. The normal corrected QT interval is considered to be <460 ms for women and <440 ms for men. Visually, the QT interval should be less than 50% of the R-R interval. Congenital long QT syndrome may be associated with a family history of sudden death or syncope, especially before the age of 40. Long QT syndrome survivors of sudden cardiac death warrant an implantable cardioverter-defibrillator. Otherwise, β-blockers are the mainstay of prevention in most cases.

A, B, E. As above.
C. IV lidocaine and oral mexiletine are among a few antiarrhythmic medications that do not prolong the QT interval, unlike quinidine, procainamide, sotalol, and amiodarone.

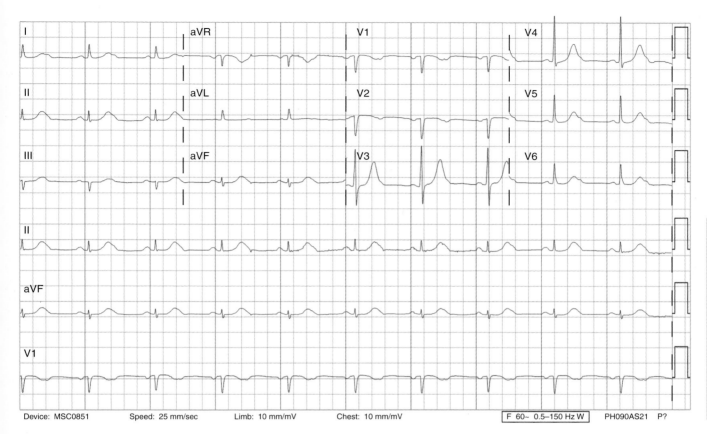

Device: MSC0851   Speed: 25 mm/sec   Limb: 10 mm/mV   Chest: 10 mm/mV   F 60~ 0.5–150 Hz W   PH090AS21 P?

15. A 56-year-old woman presents to her primary care physician complaining of 3 weeks of new fatigue. She has rarely experienced a sense of dyspnea with exertion, but denies orthopnea, chest pain, presyncope, or syncope. She takes conjugated estrogens for hot flashes after an uncomplicated hysterectomy 10 years ago. Her exam is notable for a blood pressure of 150/88 mm Hg, but is otherwise unremarkable. An ECG is done in the office. The best next step would be:

 Notes

A. Electrophysiology consultation for electrophysiology study
B. Lower extremity Doppler ultrasound
C. Initiate atenolol
D. Tilt table test
E. Stress test

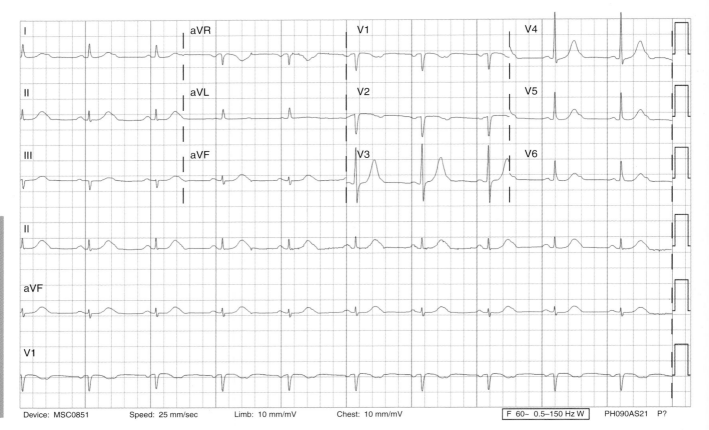

Device: MSC0851   Speed: 25 mm/sec   Limb: 10 mm/mV   Chest: 10 mm/mV   F 60~ 0.5–150 Hz W   PH090AS21   P?

15. **The answer is A: Electrophysiology consultation for electrophysiology study.** The ECG shows sinus tachycardia just above 100 bpm with second-degree 2:1 AV block. The P waves that are not conducting can be seen at the end of every T wave (most evident here in leads I, V1, and V6). Because the block is 2:1, you cannot differentiate between Mobitz I or Mobitz II second-degree AV block. Mobitz I second-degree AV block, with progressive PR lengthening before dropping a QRS, is generally considered to be intranodal (within the AV node), typically stable, and rarely requires a pacemaker (only if very symptomatic). Mobitz II second-degree AV block has a stable PR interval but manifests as random, unpredictable dropping of the QRS complexes and is infranodal, usually unstable, and often requires a pacemaker. An electrophysiology study would be indicated, given her vague complaints, to differentiate the exact level of block and need for pacemaker.

B. Though the patient takes conjugated estrogens, which can increase the possibility of venothromboembolic disease, the ECG mandates further electrophysiology evaluation first.
C. Though she is hypertensive, atenolol is contraindicated in the setting of second-degree AV block.
D. Tilt table testing is used in certain patients with syncope or presyncope, but this patient has neither complaint.
E. Though heart block and dyspnea can be associated sometimes with ischemic heart disease, the next best test in this situation is an electrophysiology evaluation.

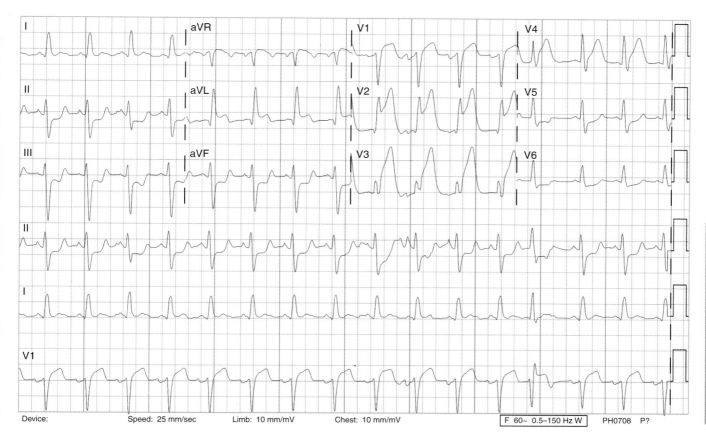

| Device: | Speed: 25 mm/sec | Limb: 10 mm/mV | Chest: 10 mm/mV | F 60~ 0.5–150 Hz W | PH0708 P? |

16. A 44-year-old man presents to the emergency department with 60 minutes of new chest fullness and diaphoresis followed by a brief loss of consciousness that began while he was carrying drywall on a job site. In the absence of any absolute contraindications, the best next step would be:

A. IV fibrinolytics under 30 minutes from arrival to the emergency department

B. Pulmonary embolus protocol CT

C. Coronary artery angiography with angioplasty with or without stenting under 90 minutes from arrival to the emergency department

D. Electrophysiology study

E. Antiinflammatory medications

 Notes

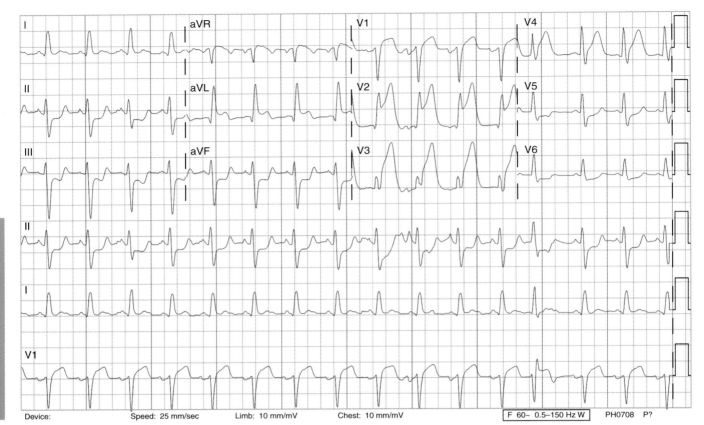

Device: Speed: 25 mm/sec   Limb: 10 mm/mV   Chest: 10 mm/mV   F 60~ 0.5–150 Hz W   PH0708   P?

16. **The answer is C: Coronary artery angiography with angioplasty with or without stenting under 90 minutes from arrival to the emergency department.** This ECG shows an acute anteroseptal injury pattern with inferolateral reciprocal ST depression, consistent with an anteroseptal ST-elevation myocardial infarction. The basic rhythm is sinus rhythm with left atrial abnormality, left ventricular hypertrophy (R wave >0.11 mV [>11 small boxes] in lead aVL) with associated left axis deviation, early precordial R/S transition (as the QRS complex transitions from negative to positive earlier than lead V3), prolonged QT, a premature junctional beat (13th beat), and with slight aberrancy (incomplete RBBB pattern by the rsR′ pattern in V1, less than 120 ms [<3 small boxes]). Coronary artery angiography with angioplasty with or without stenting within 90 minutes of arrival to the emergency department is the treatment of choice.

A. As most emergency departments do not have access to a cardiac catheterization lab, IV fibrinolytics are the second best option, and should be given within 30 minutes of arrival to the emergency department.

B, D, E. The symptoms and ST changes are not indicative of pulmonary embolus, chronic arrhythmias, or pericarditis, and therefore pulmonary embolus protocol CT, electrophysiology study, and antiinflammatory medications are not indicated. Syncope may be related to transient life-threatening VT, often associated with an acute infarction.

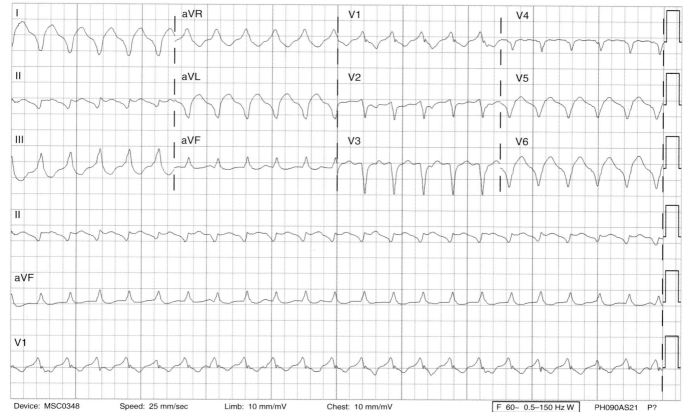

Device: MSC0348   Speed: 25 mm/sec   Limb: 10 mm/mV   Chest: 10 mm/mV   F 60~ 0.5–150 Hz W   PH090AS21   P?

17. A 70-year-old woman with a history of coronary artery disease treated with prior coronary artery stents and known right bundle branch block presents to your office for a routine visit. She complains of new mild fatigue for 1 week. Her pulse rate is 130 bpm, blood pressure is 104/76 mm Hg. Her exam is otherwise notable for canon A-waves, variable S1, and a 2/6 holosystolic murmur at the apex. Her tachycardia prompts an ECG that shows the following:

A. Sinus tachycardia with right bundle branch block and left posterior fascicular block
B. VT
C. Atrial flutter 2:1 conduction, with right bundle branch block and left posterior fascicular block
D. AVRT
E. Sinus tachycardia with left bundle branch block

✎ *Notes*

Section II CARDIOLOGY

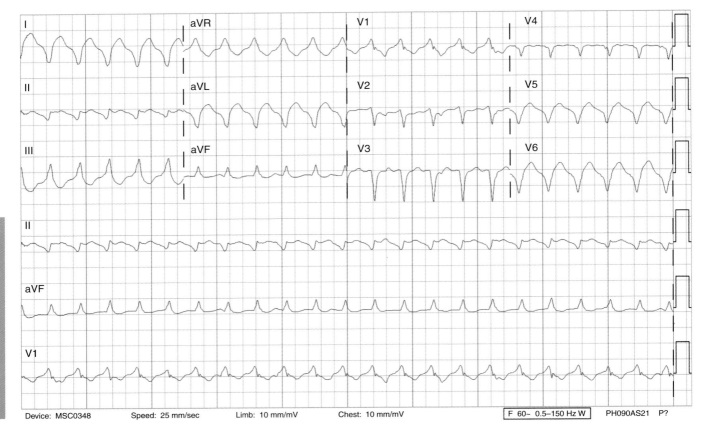

Device: MSC0348   Speed: 25 mm/sec   Limb: 10 mm/mV   Chest: 10 mm/mV   F 60~ 0.5–150 Hz W   PH090AS21   P?

17. **The answer is B: VT.** The ECG demonstrates a wide complex regular tachycardia consistent with VT. There are two other major causes of wide complex tachycardias: any supraventricular tachycardia (including sinus tachycardia) with bundle branch block aberrancy and AVRT (also known as *atrioventricular reciprocating tachycardia*). Clinically the history of coronary artery disease makes any wide complex tachycardia more likely to be VT. Importantly, hemodynamic stability does not exclude VT. Three important telemetry strip or ECG findings that confirm VT over supraventricular tachycardia with aberrancy are AV dissociation, fusion beats, and capture beats. AV dissociation is noted here with supraventricular P waves seen between the 12th and 13th beats and the 14th and 15th beats are slightly more negative deflections than on rhythm lead V1. Note these P waves are seen in lead V2, as well. With calipers, you can march these P waves both forward and backward to find other confirmatory dissociated P waves at the same atrial rate (about 70 bpm) which is slower than the VT. AV dissociation leads to a variable sounding S1 as the mitral and tricuspid valves have variable degrees of opening depending on the timing of dissociated atrial contractions. Fusion beats are QRS complexes with morphology between supraventricular conduction and ventricular conduction as the two wave

fronts meet to form one complex (not seen here). Capture beats occur when a dissociated P wave fortuitously finds the entire ventricle available for depolarization between VT beats, creating a normal native complex (not seen here). Other supporting findings to suggest VT are: an axis between –90 degrees and 180 degrees (northwest axis or far left axis); monophasic R wave in V1 (seen here); rSR′ in V1 with R′ wave taller than r; deeper S wave depth than R wave height; or QS wave in V6 (seen here). There are also other more advanced criteria called *Brugada criteria* and *lead aVR criteria*.

A. The AV dissociation excludes sinus tachycardia with right bundle branch block and left posterior fascicular block, not to mention the monophasic R wave in V1 is more consistent with VT than a typical right bundle branch block.
C. The absence of flutter waves excludes atrial flutter.
D. Wide complex AVRT occurs when there is conduction using a bypass tract, in which the reentry circuit goes down the bypass tract and up the AV node, or less commonly down the AV node, conducting with a bundle branch block aberrancy and up the bypass tract. The criteria noted in answer B favor VT and not AVRT.
E. The positive deflection in V1 excludes left bundle branch block.

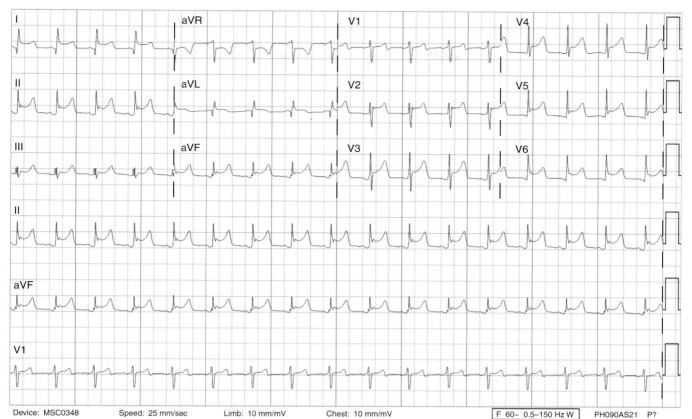

Device: MSC0348   Speed: 25 mm/sec   Limb: 10 mm/mV   Chest: 10 mm/mV   F 60~ 0.5–150 Hz W   PH090AS21 P?

18. A 46-year-old woman with a history of systemic lupus erythematosus presents with acute onset chest pain beginning 5 hours ago. It began at rest, and she reports being unable to lie flat. Her younger brother had a myocardial infarction 1 year earlier. Her exam is notable for mild distress, blood pressure 112/78 mm Hg, and pulse oximetry 93% on room air. There is a faint malar rash, slightly decreased breath sounds at the bases of her lungs, with a regular heart rhythm without murmurs or gallops. There is no lower extremity edema. Based on her ECG, the best next step is:

A. Aspirin and urgent coronary angiography with possible angioplasty and stenting
B. IV heparin and pulmonary embolus protocol CT
C. Aspirin and IV thrombolytics
D. Aspirin and an echocardiogram
E. IV heparin and eptifibatide

Notes

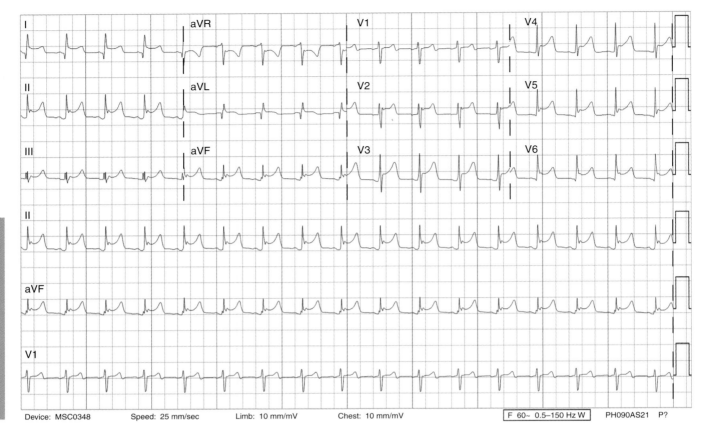

Device: MSC0348   Speed: 25 mm/sec   Limb: 10 mm/mV   Chest: 10 mm/mV   F 60~ 0.5–150 Hz W   PH090AS21   P?

18. **The answer is D: Aspirin and an echocardiogram.**
High-dose aspirin or ibuprofen is the treatment
of choice for pericarditis. In patients with a first
episode of pericarditis, regardless of cause, the
addition of colchicine appears to reduce the duration
of symptoms and the recurrence rate. There is
some suggestion that steroids are associated with a
higher recurrence rate, though they may need to be
given to treat an underlying autoimmune disease
when present, or when aspirin or nonsteroidal
antiinflammatory medications are contraindicated
or ineffective. An echocardiogram is reasonable to
assess for a pericardial effusion in this patient with
lupus. The ECG shows diffuse ST segment elevation
without reciprocal changes. ECG changes in acute
pericarditis occur in four stages, but some may be
missed. Stage one consists of concave upward ST
segment elevation and PR segment depression in
almost all leads except aVR. Stage two is when the ST
segment returns to baseline with the onset of T wave
flattening. Stage three consists of T wave inversions.

Stage four is a return to the normal ECG. Classically
the patient has worsening of symptoms when
supine and relative relief when leaning forward,
because the heart hangs from its attachment with
less approximation of the heart with the pericardial
sac walls in this position. A pericardial friction rub
is often heard as a rasping or scratching sound, but
may be absent or intermittent.

A, C, E. Though this patient has risk factors for
coronary artery disease, including lupus and the
premature family history, the ST segment elevation
is diffuse, not convex up, and not associated with
reciprocal ST segment depression. Therefore, there is
no role for coronary angiography, IV thrombolytics,
IV heparin, or eptifibatide.
B. Though the patient has chest pain with a
relatively low pulse oximetry, the ECG points toward
pericarditis as a specific cause, therefore there is no
role for pulmonary embolus protocol CT at this
point.

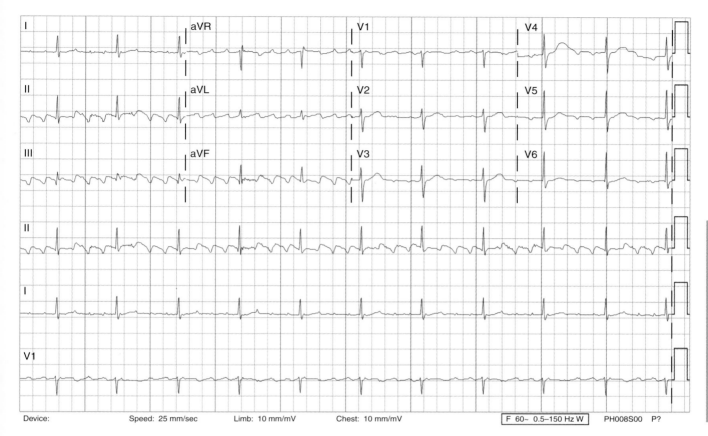

I	aVR	V1	V4
II	aVL	V2	V5
III	aVF	V3	V6

II

I

V1

Device: Speed: 25 mm/sec   Limb: 10 mm/mV   Chest: 10 mm/mV   F 60~ 0.5–150 Hz W   PH008S00   P?

19. A 51-year-old man with non-insulin–dependent diabetes, hypertension, hyperlipidemia, and chronic obstructive pulmonary disease (COPD) presents for a physical in order to apply for a life insurance policy. His medications include metformin, atenolol, hydrochlorothiazide, and tiotropium inhaler. An ECG is performed. The best next step is:

 Notes

A. Aspirin
B. Increase atenolol
C. Dronedarone
D. Amiodarone
E. Warfarin

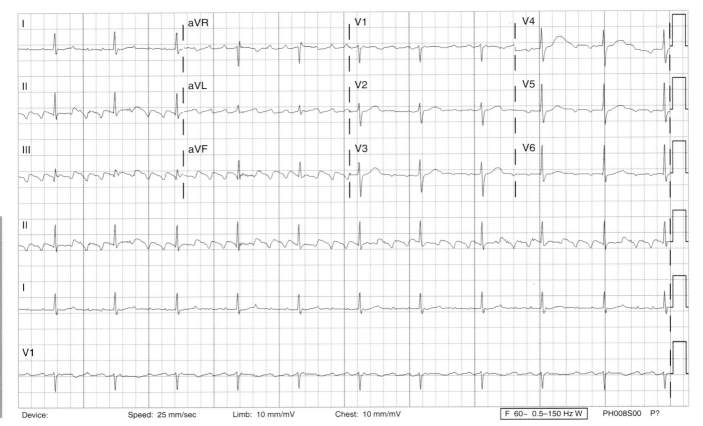

Device: Speed: 25 mm/sec   Limb: 10 mm/mV   Chest: 10 mm/mV   F 60~ 0.5–150 Hz W   PH008S00   P?

19. **The answer is E: Warfarin.** The ECG shows atrial flutter with 4:1 conduction. Warfarin is indicated given his history of diabetes and hypertension. Atrial flutter is a reentrant atrial arrhythmia which typically has an atrial rate of between 250 and 350 bpm. If this patient was not already taking atenolol, the atrial flutter may have conducted 2:1, resulting in a heart rate of about 150 bpm, which may make seeing the flutter waves more difficult. The most common form of atrial flutter has dominant negative flutter deflections in the inferior leads and positive flutter deflections in lead V1 due to counterclockwise rotation within the right atrium, passing through the cavotricuspid isthmus. Generally atrial flutter is acutely treated like atrial fibrillation. If unstable, cardioversion is indicated. If tachycardic, IV or oral rate controlling agents can be offered such as non-dihydropyridine calcium channel blockers, β-blockers, and less commonly digitalis. Anticoagulation decisions are similar to those for atrial fibrillation, though there are less data. Lastly, catheter based ablative therapies can be offered, particularly when the atrial flutter is counterclockwise involving the cavotricuspid isthmus, such as this.

A. Aspirin would be insufficient because he has two risk factors for thromboembolism: diabetes and hypertension (CHADS2 score of 2).
B. Increasing his atenolol dose would not be necessary given he is already adequately rate controlled at rest.
C. Amiodarone or dronedarone are antiarrhythmic agents which should not be started without anticoagulation in this patient.

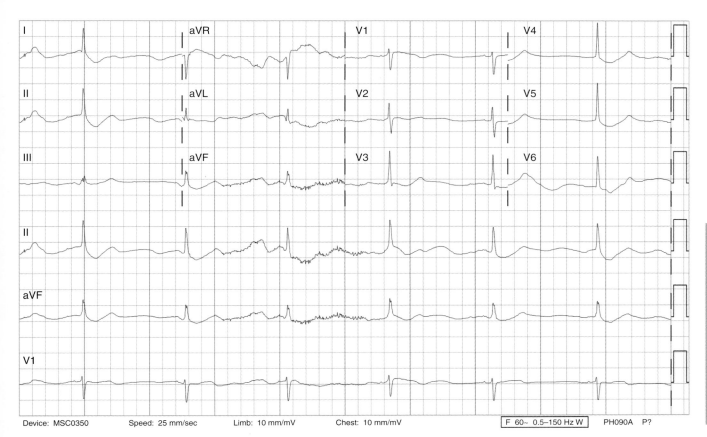

Device: MSC0350   Speed: 25 mm/sec   Limb: 10 mm/mV   Chest: 10 mm/mV   F 60~ 0.5–150 Hz W   PH090A   P?

20. A 77-year-old woman with paroxysmal atrial fibrillation, diabetes, and breast cancer recently had her diltiazem increased and digoxin added 3 weeks earlier for rapid ventricular rates. Over the last several weeks, she has had progressive fatigue, anorexia, and several near-syncopal episodes. An ECG is performed in the office. Which of the following statements is most true regarding her diagnosis?

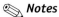 **Notes**

A. There is complete heart block.
B. Coronary angiography should be urgently performed.
C. Ventricular arrhythmias are uncommon.
D. Vision changes are common.
E. Glucagon should be given.

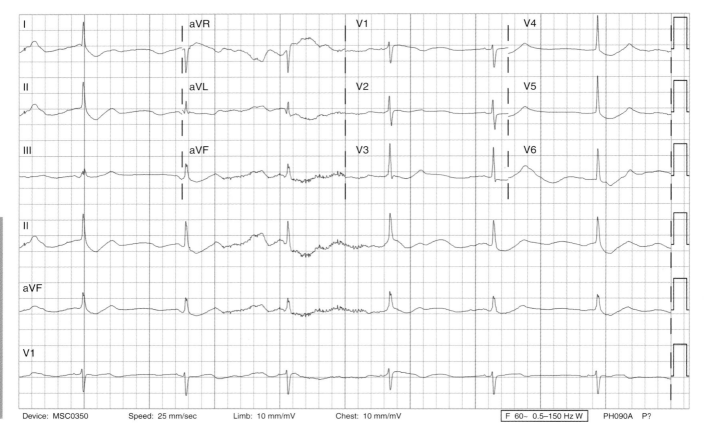

Device: MSC0350   Speed: 25 mm/sec   Limb: 10 mm/mV   Chest: 10 mm/mV   F 60~ 0.5–150 Hz W   PH090A   P?

20. **The answer is D: Vision changes are common.** This ECG reveals sinus bradycardia with a rate below 40 bpm, with ST segment changes consistent with digitalis effect. The constellation of fatigue, anorexia, and presyncope combined with this ECG revealing significant bradycardia raises the concern for digitalis toxicity. Vision changes are relatively common, including color vision complaints, scotomas and, rarely, blindness. With chronic toxicity, serum digitalis levels do not correlate with toxicity as asymptomatic patients can have elevated levels, and toxic patients could have therapeutic levels. Medications such as diltiazem, verapamil, amiodarone, and quinidine can increase digitalis levels, as can renal failure. Arrhythmias are common, including bradyarrhythmias (including complete heart block) due to excessive parasympathetic tone, junctional arrhythmias, ventricular ectopy, and VTs, including biventricular tachycardia, and classically, atrial fibrillation or flutter with AV block. ST segment

changes from digitalis effect are a normal J point (the transition point between the QRS complex and the ST segment) followed immediately by a sagging or scooped ST segment. ECG digitalis effect alone does not indicate toxicity.

A. Though complete heart block is associated with digitalis toxicity, this ECG shows P waves before each QRS complex, excluding complete heart block here.
B. The ST segment changes are not typical of ischemia, but rather digitalis effect.
C. Ventricular arrhythmias are common with digitalis toxicity, especially in patients with preexisting heart disease.
E. Glucagon can be used as an antidote for β-blocker and calcium channel blocker toxicity. However, the constellation of symptoms and ECG findings is more concerning for digitalis toxicity, therefore digoxin immune Fab should be given.

Section III
RADIOLOGY

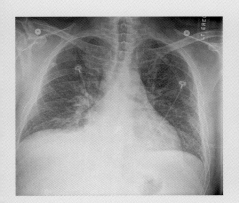
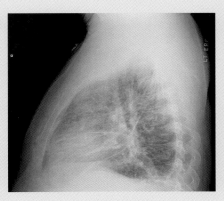
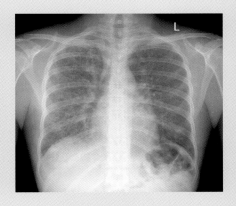

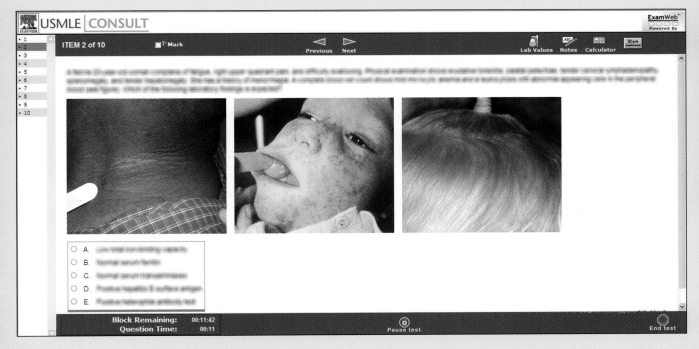

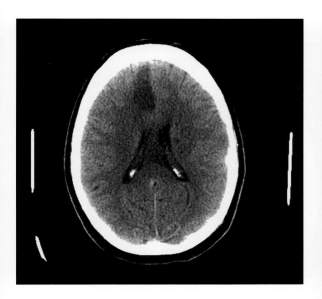
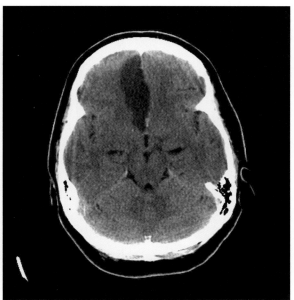

1. A 69-year-old woman with a history of poorly controlled hypertension and type 2 diabetes mellitus presented with a history of left-sided weakness and sensory deficit predominantly involving the lower limb, with hypobulia. The computed tomography (CT) scan is above. The most likely cause of the above finding is:

A. Hypertensive intracranial hemorrhage
B. Atherosclerotic occlusion of the right middle cerebral artery (MCA)
C. Atherosclerotic occlusion of the right anterior cerebral artery (ACA)
D. Ischemic infarction secondary to hypoperfusion

✎ *Notes*

ACA Infarct

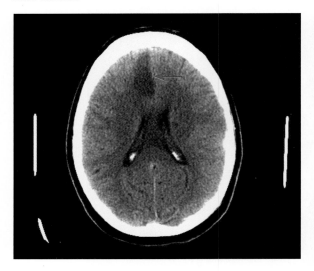 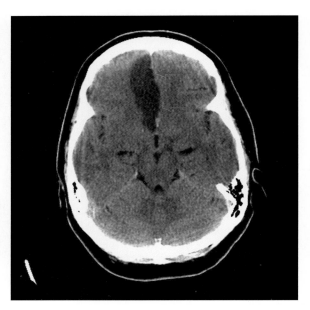

1. The answer is C: Atherosclerotic occlusion of the anterior cerebral artery (ACA). There is hypodensity (arrows) with mild mass effect involving the paramedian right frontal lobe. This is consistent with an ACA territory acute ischemic infarct. The most common cause of an ischemic ACA territory infarct is atherosclerotic occlusion, typically at the A2 origin. The patient's history of hypertension and type 2 diabetes predispose her to atherosclerotic disease.

A. The patient's history does put her at risk for hypertensive intracranial hemorrhage. However, this would present as a hyperdensity, most commonly involving the basal ganglia, followed by the cerebellum and pons.

B. The appearance is consistent with an ischemic infarct due to arterial occlusion. However, the territory involved is not consistent with the territory covered by the MCA.

D. The appearance is consistent with an ischemic infarction. However, infarcts related to hypoperfusion typically present at the border zones between vascular territories.

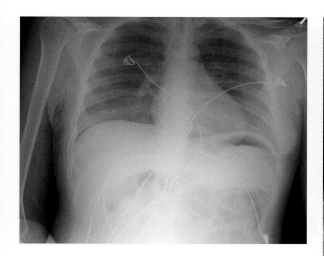

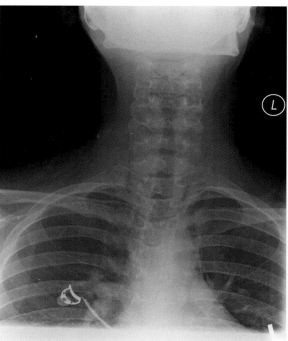

2. A 20-year-old woman with a history of asthma presents to the emergency department complaining of chest and neck discomfort. Her chest x-ray (left) and neck x-ray (right) are shown above.

Which of the following is the correct diagnosis?

A. Pneumomediastinum
B. Pneumothorax
C. Pneumoperitoneum
D. Hyperinflation without extra pulmonary air
E. Pneumothorax and pneumomediastinum

✎ Notes

Pneumomediastinum with Asthma

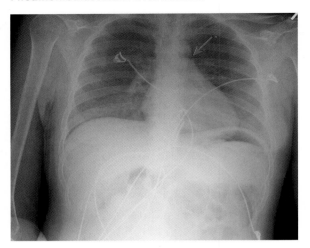

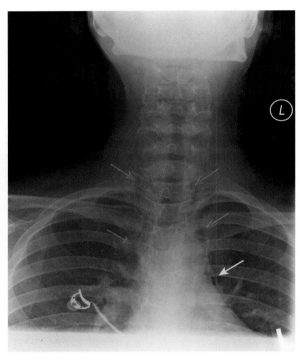

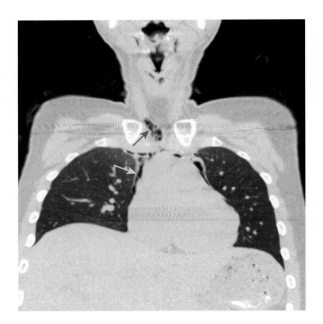

treatment in this situation. A chest x-ray is done to be certain there is no pneumothorax, which may require treatment with a chest tube.

The chest x-ray shows faint lucent streaks of air along the borders of the superior mediastinum (yellow arrows). The neck x-ray shows more obvious lucent streaks extending from the superior mediastinum into the soft tissue planes of the neck (red arrows). In this case, a chest CT (above right) was also performed, confirming mediastinal air dissecting into the neck, although CT evaluation is not mandatory in this benign clinical situation. Had the patient been vomiting or had she swallowed something sharp, there would be reason to suspect an esophageal tear, and a Gastrografin swallow and chest CT would be required.

B, E. No pneumothorax is visible on the chest x-ray. The lung apices are also well visualized on the neck x-ray, with no evidence of pneumothorax.
C. There is no evidence of pneumoperitoneum, which typically appears as a lucent zone of air beneath the right hemidiaphragm. The air seen beneath this patient's left hemidiaphragm represents the normal gastric air bubble.
D. There is no evidence of hyperinflation despite the history of asthma. The lung volumes appear normal with no hyperlucency and no flattening of the diaphragm.

2. The answer is A: Pneumomediastinum. Spontaneous pneumomediastinum may occur in any patient with coughing or straining, but it is more common among asthmatics. The cause is believed to be spontaneous rupture of a small bleb along the medial pleural surface, close to the mediastinum. This patient's symptoms of sudden onset of chest discomfort with chest and neck tightness is a typical clinical manifestation of spontaneous pneumomediastinum, which requires no

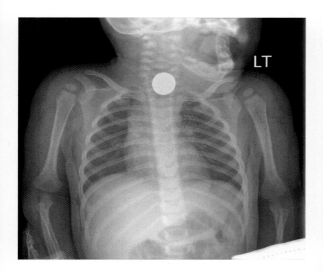

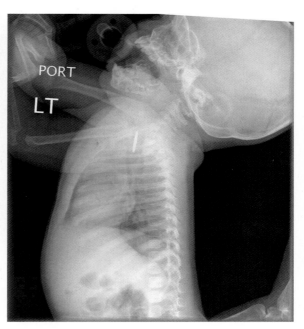

3. A mother reports to the pediatrician with her 9-month-old son with a chief complaint of refusal to feed today and increased drooling. The infant is inconsolably crying, making auscultation of the lungs difficult, but appears dyspneic, and between cries the physician hears stridor. The child is transferred to the nearest emergency department and anteroposterior (AP) and lateral chest radiographs are obtained. Which of the following statements is true?

A. Based on the radiographic findings, a bronchoscopy should be performed immediately.
B. The right lung is hyperinflated relative to the left.
C. In the setting of a suspected foreign body within the airway, if radiographs are normal, bronchoscopy is not indicated.
D. Dyspnea and stridor can occur in children when a foreign body is within the esophagus.
E. Low-dose CT of the thorax is not helpful in evaluation for foreign bodies within both the esophagus and airways.

✎ *Notes*

Foreign Body in Esophagus (Coin)

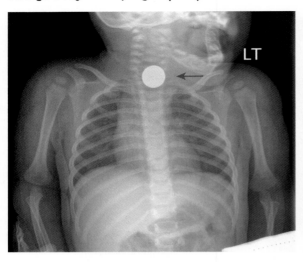

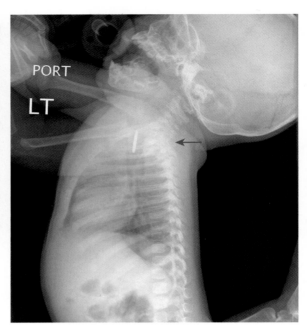

3. **The answer is D: Dyspnea and stridor can occur in children when a foreign body is within the esophagus.** This infant presents with fairly typical signs and symptoms of foreign body ingestion/aspiration. The radiographs confirm the presence of a circular metallic foreign body at the level of the thoracic inlet, posterior to the trachea on the lateral view, and in a coronal orientation (arrows); thus, impacted within the esophagus. A clue that the presumed coin is in the esophagus on the AP radiograph is its coronal orientation *(en face),* because a coin-shaped object would favor a sagittal orientation *(en profil)* within the trachea (due to the incomplete posterior cartilaginous rings of the trachea). Foreign bodies within the esophagus can have mass effect on the posterior trachea and induce dyspnea and stridor, especially at the thoracic inlet, often confounding the clinical presentation.

Foreign body aspiration/ingestion is a common cause of respiratory and gastrointestinal (GI) malady in the pediatric population. Potential complications of esophageal foreign bodies include impaction, laceration, and perforation. Aspirated or ingested foreign bodies can manifest with both acute and chronic symptoms and signs. The preferred method of extraction of impacted esophageal foreign bodies is through endoscopy, with overall a minimal complication rate.

A. Had the foreign body been within the trachea on the lateral view, an immediate bronchoscopy for retrieval would have been indicated.

B. A foreign body that is aspirated can often obstruct an airway distal to the trachea and create a ball-valve effect, resulting in hyperinflation of lung distal to the obstruction. Of course, neither lung is hyperinflated in this case. However, if aspiration, as opposed to ingestion, were still a consideration, additional lateral decubitus views could be obtained. Normally in the lateral decubitus position, the side down will be less inflated due to the weight of the body; but, in the ball-valve obstruction type scenario, the side down with the obstruction may be hyperinflated.

C. Coins are probably the most commonly swallowed foreign body, but anything small is a potential ingestion/aspiration hazard for children, especially under the age of 2, and most airway foreign bodies are not radiopaque. Therefore, in a child with acute respiratory symptoms or who is unstable, bronchoscopy should be performed irrespective of negative radiographs.

E. If the child's symptoms are of a more chronic nature, low-dose CT of the thorax, with potential for CT bronchography, is certainly indicated to identify the location of a potential esophageal or airway foreign body and direct the endoscopist/bronchoscopist.

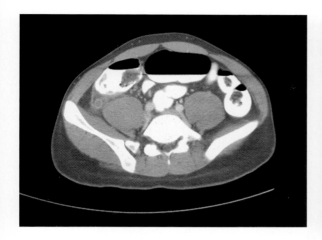
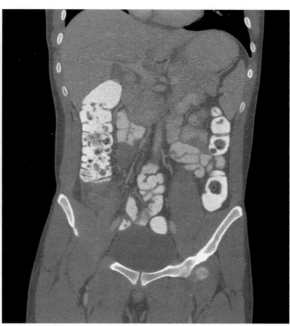

4. A 23-year-old man presents to the emergency department with fever, nausea, and vomiting and is found to have diffuse abdominal tenderness and a leukocytosis. A CT of the abdomen is performed. Which of the statements regarding the CT findings is correct?

A. The pericecal fat is normal in density.
B. The appendix is abnormally dilated, and its wall is abnormally enhancing.
C. This appendix is likely to be compressible on ultrasound.
D. There is an appendicolith.
E. There is strong evidence of appendiceal perforation.

✎ *Notes*

Acute Appendicitis

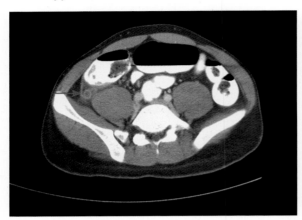

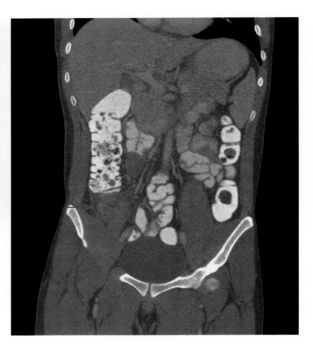

4. **The answer is B: The appendix is abnormally dilated and its wall is abnormally enhancing.** This is a fairly typical presentation for appendicitis. On the images above, there is a dilated, retrocecal appendix (red arrows) with avid wall enhancement and marked periappendiceal fat infiltration, all findings supporting a diagnosis of acute appendicitis. On CT the appendix should be less than 7 mm in diameter. A fluid-filled appendix without intraluminal air or contrast (if administered), and cecal inflammation can add to the suspicion.

Acute appendicitis is due to luminal obstruction, usually at the ostia (by an appendicolith or hypertrophied Peyer patches) and a superimposed infection. Associated complications include perforation with pneumoperitoneum and periappendiceal abscess formation. Treatment is surgical resection, if the lesion is not perforated or is minimally perforated,

and percutaneous drainage if a well-formed abscess develops in the setting of perforation. In certain patient populations, such as pregnant and pediatric patients, ultrasound is a preferred initial imaging modality in suspected appendicitis to avoid irradiation.

A. As above, the pericecal fat is abnormal in density.
C. Additional sonographic findings suggestive of appendicitis include a noncompressible appendix, tenderness while scanning the appendix, and appendiceal wall hyperemia on Doppler analysis.
D. An appendicolith is a calcified concretion that forms within the lumen of the appendix, and when present is highly suggestive of appendicitis. In this case, there is no appendicolith.
E. On the selected images, there is no pneumo-peritoneum or well-formed periappendiceal abscess to suggest perforation.

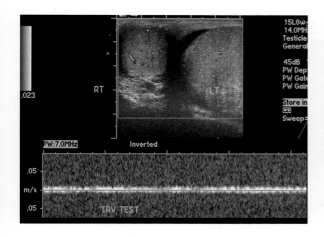
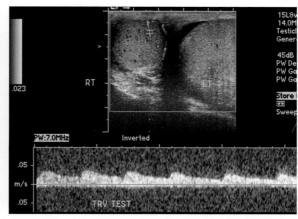
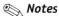

5. A 14-year-old boy presents to the emergency department with severe left scrotal pain. While he had been experiencing pain off and on for about a week, the pain is now much worse and has been constant for about 3 hours. An ultrasound is ordered. Which of the following statements is true?

A. Both testes are symmetric in size.

B. While there is no waveform in the sampled area of the left testicle, there is evidence of blood flow based on the power Doppler analysis.

C. The sonographic findings are suggestive of neoplasm.

D. If the involved testicle is found to be viable, the preferred surgical treatment is 100% effective in preventing recurrence.

E. No further imaging is necessary.

✎ *Notes*

Testicular Torsion

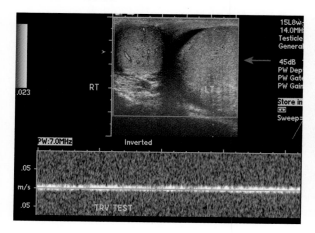 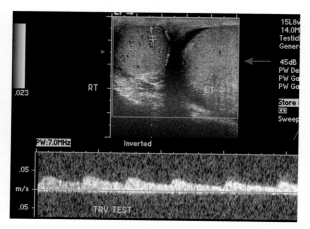

5. **The answer is E: No further imaging is necessary.**
The sonographic images are diagnostic of left testicular torsion, and no further imaging should delay prompt intervention. The left testicle is markedly larger than the right, and there is no blood flow demonstrated on both power and spectral Doppler analysis (arrows).

Testicular torsion occurs when the testis and spermatic cord twist, either spontaneously or secondary to trauma, causing the vascular pedicle to twist as well and resulting in vascular compromise. Viability of the testis depends on the degree of torsion and the time of onset of pain to intervention, with an 80% chance of salvage within 6 hours and a 0% chance after 12 hours. There is a bimodal peak age of incidence in infants and adolescents. Up to 50% of patients report a history of similar symptoms resolving spontaneously.

A. The left testicle is markedly larger than the right.
B. There is no blood flow demonstrated on both power and spectral Doppler analysis.
C. There is no neoplasm by sonographic findings.
D. While manual detorsion can be attempted, surgery is the definitive treatment, and if the testicle is found to be viable, orchidopexy is helpful in preventing recurrent torsion but not failsafe. If the testicle is not viable at surgery, it should be removed, because the blood-testis barrier may potentially break down, allowing the patient to develop immunity against his own sperm, thus lowering his fertility (the so-called antisperm antibody theory).

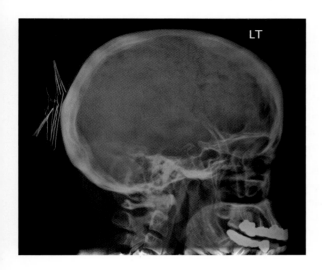

6. A 60-year-old woman presents to her primary care physician with complaints of intermittent mild bone pain, especially in the back. She has lost weight since her last visit. She is found to be mildly anemic and to have mild renal insufficiency on laboratory tests. Further testing of the patient's urine reveals the presence of Bence Jones proteins. She is sent for magnetic resonance imaging (MRI) of the spine. She informs the MRI technologist that she long ago had a piece of metal stuck in her eye after a car accident. A lateral radiograph of the skull is performed to evaluate for metallic foreign body in the orbits prior to the MRI. Which of the following statements is true?

A. The patient likely has elevated serum calcium.
B. There is intraorbital metal, an absolute contraindication to an MRI.
C. Findings on the radiograph suggest a process involving overactive osteoblasts and suppressed osteoclasts.
D. If this disease involves the lumbar spine, MRI to be performed is not sensitive in identifying lesions.
E. The patient's prognosis is favorable.

Myeloma Involving the Calvarium

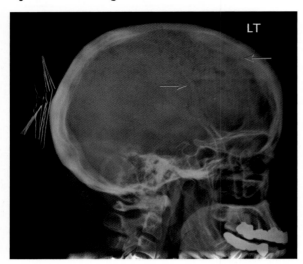

6. The answer is A: The patient likely has elevated serum calcium. The lateral radiograph of the skull shows multiple, well-defined, lytic lesions throughout the calvarium (red arrows), with a "punched-out" appearance, which, especially with the clinical information provided, are highly likely due to myeloma. There are multiple lesions; therefore the stage of the disease is more likely to be advanced, and the patient likely has elevated serum calcium due to the osseous destruction. Myeloma is a monoclonal plasma cell malignancy arising from the bone marrow. Myeloma is the most common primary bone neoplasm. Common sites of involvement of myeloma include the spine, ribs, pelvis, skull, femur, and humerus. Myeloma is primarily treated with chemotherapy.

B. There are no metallic foreign bodies within the orbits on the radiograph provided, so without any other obvious contraindications, the patient is safe to have the MRI.
C. The neoplastic plasma cells in myeloma release cytokines that increase osteoclastic activity and suppress osteoblastic activity, ultimately leading to the lucent lesions with little to no associated sclerosis (i.e., new bone formation).
D. MRI is the best imaging tool when evaluating for any marrow-replacing process, such as myeloma or metastases, the two most common bone malignancies in adults. Therefore the MRI to be performed in this case would be highly sensitive for disease involving the spine.
E. Despite therapeutic advancements, myeloma continues to be a fatal disease, especially at an advanced stage.

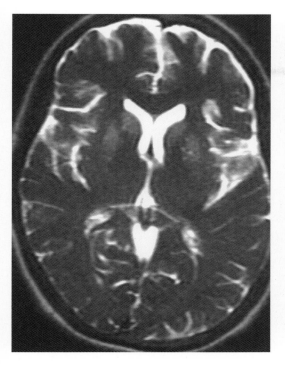

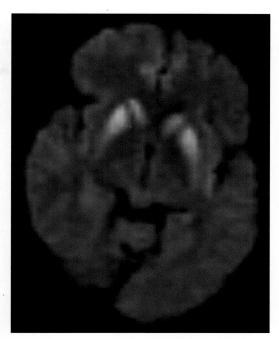

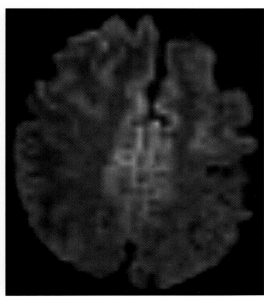

7. A 48-year-old man presented to his primary care physician with a 6-month history of gradually increased awareness of sudden random muscular jerking. His wife reports that his thinking seems to be more clouded and there are personality changes. The MRI demonstrated symmetric signal abnormality within the cerebral cortex, caudate heads, and putamen on the T2 and diffusion-weighted images. The most likely diagnosis is:

A. Multiple sclerosis
B. Encephalitis
C. Creutzfeldt-Jakob disease (CJD)
D. Multi-infarct dementia

 Notes

Creutzfeldt-Jakob Disease (CJD)

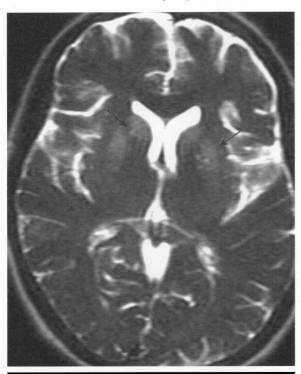

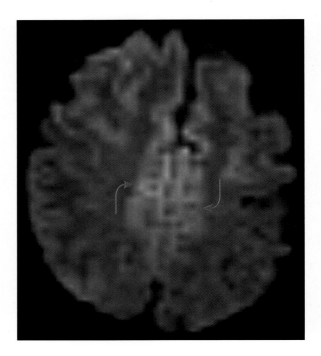

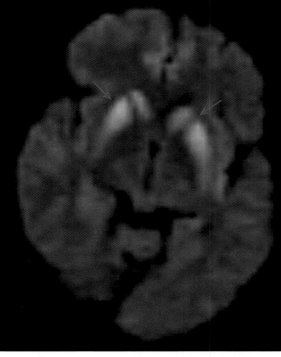

7. The answer is C: Creutzfeldt-Jakob disease (CJD).
The pattern of hyperintense signal on T2 (top left) and diffusion-weighted imaging (bottom left, top right) within the bilateral putamen and caudate head (straight arrows) as well as the bilateral paramedian gyri (curved arrows) is classic for CJD. The three major categories of CJD are sporadic, hereditary, and acquired. The sporadic form is the most common, accounting for at least 85% of cases. The hereditary form will have a family history of the disease and test positive for a genetic mutation. The acquired form demonstrates several variant subtypes, with variable symptoms and course of the disease. The sporadic and variant types of CJD are more likely to demonstrate signal abnormality within the thalamus, the so-called pulvinar sign.

A. Multiple sclerosis should demonstrate T2 signal abnormality involving the periventricular and subcortical white matter, not the gray matter as seen here.
B. Encephalitis should demonstrate T2 signal abnormality involving both the gray and white matter and should not be symmetric.
D. Multi-infarct dementia should demonstrate multiple areas of old infarcts with volume loss and gliosis. While there may be focal areas of diffusion restriction representing acute infarcts, it would not demonstrate the symmetry seen here.

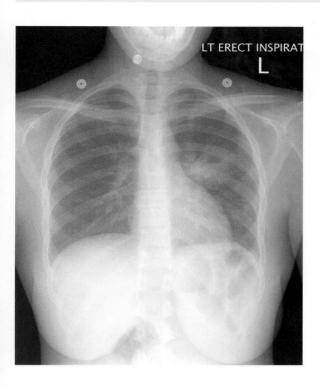

8. An 18-year-old woman presents to the emergency department complaining of chest discomfort. On physical examination, she is mildly tachypneic and tachycardic, with a fever of 101° F. Her past medical history is significant for a seizure disorder. Her chest x-ray is above.

  What is the most likely diagnosis?
  A. Fungal pneumonia
  B. Squamous cell carcinoma of the lung
  C. Lung abscess
  D. Pulmonary embolus
  E. Wegener granulomatosis

9. What additional studies are indicated at this time?

  A. CT scan of the chest
  B. CT scan of the chest, abdomen, and pelvis
  C. MRI scan of the chest
  D. MRI scan of the brain
  E. Ventilation/perfusion scan of the lungs

Lung Abscess

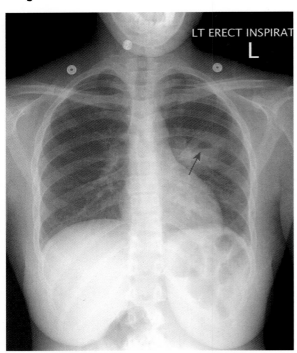

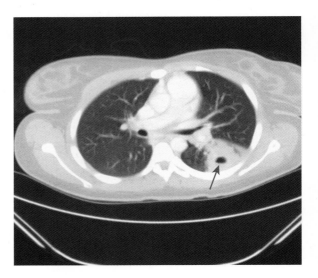

8. **The answer is C: Lung abscess.** The chest x-ray shows a 6-cm masslike structure in the left lung. The mass has typical features of an abscess, including an area of central cavitation with an air-fluid level (arrow). The patient's underlying seizure disorder puts her at significant risk of aspiration, which was the cause of this infection.

A, B, E. The differential diagnosis of cavitary lung masses also includes fungal infections, squamous cell tumors, and Wegener granulomatosis, among other less likely etiologies. However, the patient's profile, including her young age and her history of seizure disorder, render these other diagnoses unlikely. **D.** Pulmonary embolus may present with chest discomfort, tachypnea, and tachycardia but would not produce a large cavitary mass. Most patients with pulmonary embolus have normal chest x-rays, but the most common abnormalities would be focal atelectasis and small pleural effusion.

9. **The correct answer is A: CT scan of the chest.** Chest CT is indicated to confirm the x-ray findings, to evaluate for possible additional abnormalities, and to establish a baseline appearance for follow-up comparison. A representative image from the CT study (above) confirms a large mass with central necrosis and air-fluid level (arrow) in the superior segment of the left lower lung. No additional abscesses are present.

B, D. There is no indication to perform additional imaging of the abdomen, pelvis, or brain at this time. **E.** As there is no reason to suspect pulmonary embolism, there is no indication for ventilation/perfusion scanning.

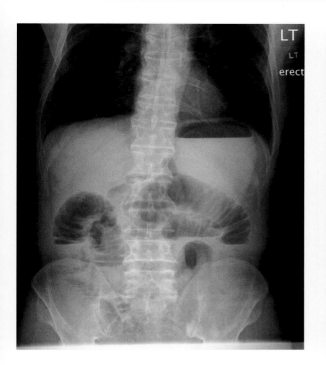

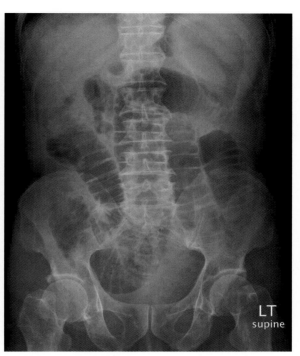

10. A 50-year-old man presents to the emergency department with abdominal bloating, nausea, vomiting, and no bowel movement in 4 days. Past surgical history is significant for appendectomy as a young adult. On physical exam, the abdomen is distended, and there is a paucity of bowel sounds, but there is no rebound tenderness. The patient's vital signs are stable and laboratory tests are normal. While waiting for a surgical consult, abdominal radiographs are performed. Which of the following statements is correct?

A. There is a large bowel obstruction.
B. There is a small bowel obstruction.
C. There are signs of vascular compromise.
D. CT of the abdomen is unnecessary.
E. Tumor is the most likely etiology.

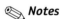 *Notes*

Small Bowel Obstruction

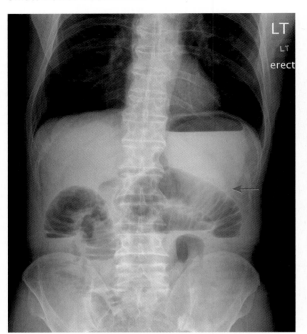

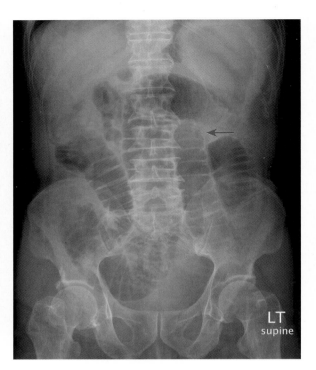

10. **The answer is B: There is a small bowel obstruction.**
The patient presents with symptoms concerning for
bowel obstruction. The radiographs are supportive of
a high-grade small bowel obstruction. The colon is not
visualized, and the dilated loops are clearly small bowel
(arrows), as evidenced by the presence of valvulae
conniventes.

Radiographic findings supportive of small bowel
obstruction include dilated small bowel loops,
presence of valvulae conniventes, multiple air-fluid
levels on erect or decubitus views, and a relative
absence of air and stool throughout the large bowel.
The first course of action should be decompression via
placement of a nasogastric tube. Given the fluid-filled
stomach, the patient will very much appreciate this
procedure. Complications of small bowel obstruction
include bowel strangulation, perforation, and sepsis.

Prognosis of an uncomplicated obstruction is good.
A trial of conservative management with bowel rest,
decompression, and hydration may prove helpful in
low grade obstructions.

A. The colon is not visualized, and the dilated loops
are clearly small bowel, as evidenced by the presence
of valvulae conniventes.
C. There are no obvious radiographic findings
of potential vascular compromise (e.g., volvulus,
pneumatosis, pneumoperitoneum).
D. CT of the abdomen is indicated in this scenario in
order to help identify the cause, grade the severity, and
offer information for surgical planning.
E. The most common cause of small bowel
obstruction is adhesions, followed by hernias, and
then tumors.

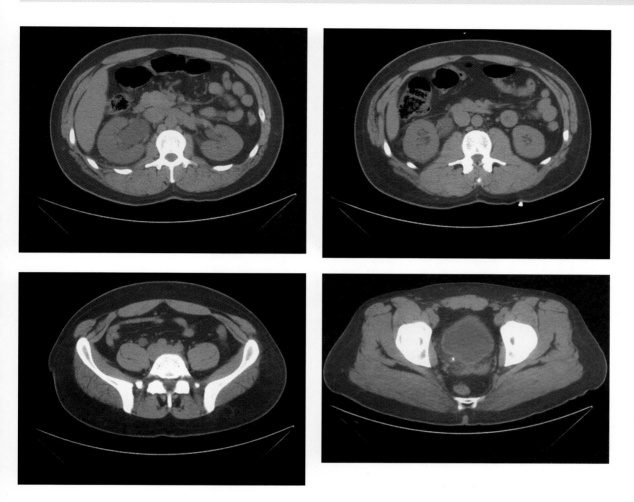

11. A 23-year-old man presents to the emergency department with severe colicky right flank pain, which radiates to the groin. He is afebrile, and his vital signs are stable. A urinalysis reveals hematuria. A CT of the abdomen (above) and pelvis (p. 196) is obtained. Which of the following statements is true?

A. Intravenous (IV) contrast should have been administered.
B. The cause of pain is most likely musculoskeletal in origin.
C. This disease process is more common in women.
D. Radiographs are considered sufficient to make this diagnosis.
E. There is obstructive uropathy on the right.

✎ *Notes*

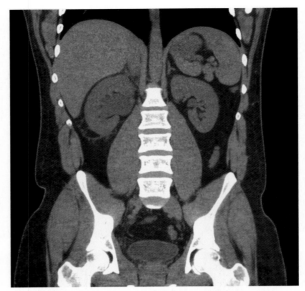

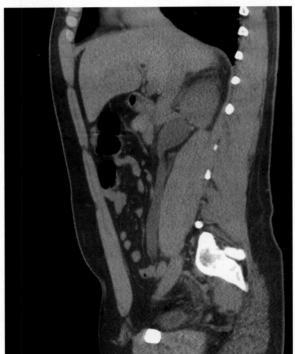

Obstructive Urolithiasis (additional figures on p. 198)

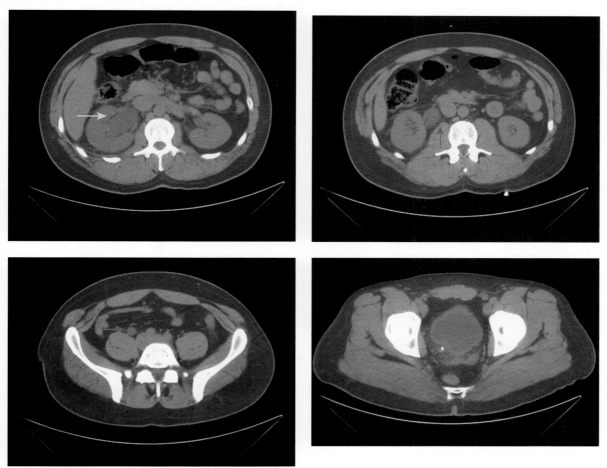

11. **The answer is E: There is obstructive uropathy on the right.** The CT images provided demonstrate an obstructing calculus in the right ureterovesicular junction (red arrow), under 10 mm in size. There is resulting hydroureter (blue arrow), hydronephrosis (yellow arrow), enlargement of the right kidney, and right perinephric fat standing.

Urolithiasis should be considered very likely in patients who present with acute colicky flank pain that radiates to the groin. Distal ureteral calculi less than 10 mm in size can pass spontaneously. Ultrasound is the preferred initial imaging test in suspected urolithiasis in pregnant patients. In the absence of complications such as renal failure, anuria, or urosepsis, hydration and analgesia with oral pain medications is usually the initial treatment in patients with small stones.

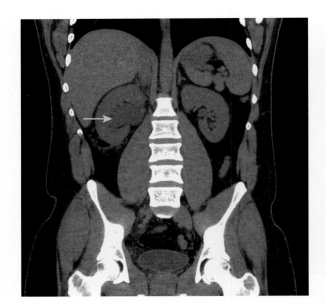

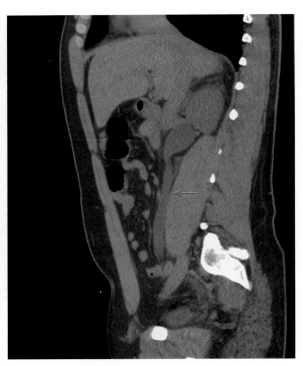

A. In adults with suspected urolithiasis with acute symptoms, CT of the abdomen without contrast is the preferred study of choice. The sensitivity and specificity of a noncontrast CT in identifying ureterolithiasis are 95% and 98%, respectively. Because a majority of calculi are hyperdense on CT, a urographic CT phase with IV contrast is rarely necessary and usually reserved for special scenarios, such as identifying radiolucent stones in patients on idinavir (a protease inhibitor).

B. Besides the ureteral stone being an obvious cause of the patient's symptoms, there is no evidence provided on the CT images that there is a musculoskeletal abnormality.

C. Urolithiasis is three times more common in men.

D. Despite old teachings that 90% of renal and ureteral calculi can be seen on radiographs, and the fact that most stones are composed of calcium, comparison studies with CT have shown that the sensitivity of radiographs is actually about 60%.

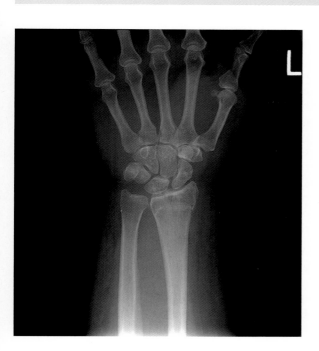

12. A 65-year-old woman presents to her primary care physician after tripping in her driveway and is complaining of left wrist pain and swelling. She is referred to the local imaging center for radiographs of the left wrist, and she returns to her doctor with one radiograph from the study. Which of the following statements is true?

A. No other radiographic views are necessary in this case.
B. This is not the expected location of injury, given the patient's age.
C. When the patient fell, she likely landed on the palm of her dorsiflexed hand.
D. Most of these injuries require surgery.
E. An underlying advanced inflammatory arthropathy predisposed the patient to this injury.

Distal Radial Fracture

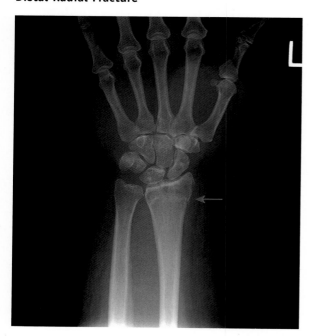

12. **The answer is C: When the patient fell, she likely landed on the palm of her dorsiflexed hand.** This patient has suffered a fracture of her left distal radius (red arrow). The single posteroanterior (PA) radiograph shows the comminuted impacted fracture, which has an intraarticular component extending to the radiocarpal joint.

In people approximately 40 years old and older, the most common fracture at the wrist that results from a "fall on an outstretched hand" (FOOSH) when the hand is dorsiflexed is the distal radial fracture. There are many types of distal radial fractures, the majority given eponyms, and the most common being the Colles fracture, in which there is a transverse fracture through the distal radius and apex volar angulation. Colles fractures tend to occur in osteoporotic bone. Distal radial fractures are largely due to axial compression with variable tensile forces, especially in the setting of FOOSH.

A. While there appears to be no displacement or angulation on this single view, at least a lateral view is necessary to fully characterize the fracture and guide therapy.
B. In people approximately 40 years old and older, the most common fracture at the wrist that results from a FOOSH when the hand is dorsiflexed is the distal radius fracture.
D. Most distal radial fractures are treated with reduction and immobilization, and surgery is not needed.
E. There is no evidence on the radiograph of an underlying advanced inflammatory arthropathy, such as joint space narrowing, erosions, or juxtaarticular osteopenia.

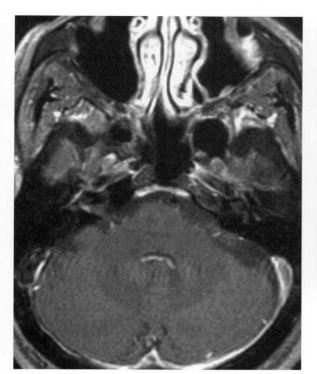
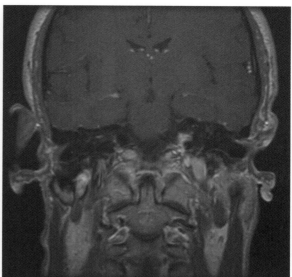

13. A 47-year-old woman presented to her primary care physician's office with a 2-week history of increasing weakness of her right face and noticed yesterday that she could not fully close her eyelid. Imaging was obtained. The most likely etiology for the patient's symptoms is:

A. Facial nerve schwannoma
B. Bell palsy (facial neuritis)
C. Vestibular schwannoma
D. Acute erosive otomastoiditis

 Notes

Bell Palsy

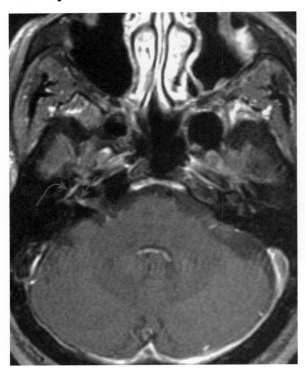

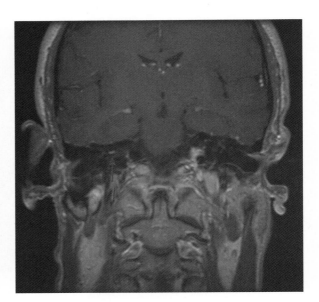

13. **The answer is B: Bell palsy (facial neuritis).**
Postcontrast T1-weighted imaging demonstrated enhancement of the right facial nerve that included the tympanic segment and geniculate ganglion (curved arrow) with extension into the internal auditory canal (IAC) (straight arrows). The facial nerve is broken down into anatomic segments: the meatal segment is from the brain stem to the IAC; the labyrinthine segment is from the fundus of the IAC to facial hiatus; the tympanic segment is from the geniculate ganglion to the pyramidal eminence; the mastoid segment is from the pyramidal process to the stylomastoid foramen; and the extratemporal segment is from the stylomastoid foramen to the pes anserinus.

The facial nerve may demonstrate mild enhancement normally up to and within the geniculate ganglion and tympanic segment, but enhancement should never extend more proximally through to the labyrinthine segment and into the IAC. The appearance of thin wispy enhancement extending into the fundus of the IAC is consistent with Bell palsy.

A. Facial nerve schwannoma can be a cause of slowly progressive facial weakness rather than the acute presentation seen in this patient. It typically presents as a nodular enhancing mass anywhere along the nerve course. The symptoms would depend on the segment of nerve involved.
C. Vestibular schwannoma typically presents in a patient with sensorineural hearing loss demonstrating nodular enhancement within the IAC and frequently extension into the cerebellopontine angle with widening of the porus acusticus.
D. Acute erosive otomastoiditis should present with additional symptoms of pain, fever, and possibly conductive hearing loss. There should be abnormal signal and enhancement within the mastoid air cells, not seen in these images.

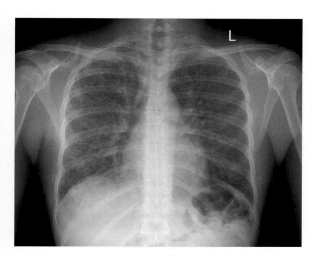

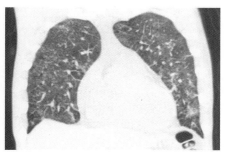

14. A 23-year-old man presents to the emergency department with symptoms of malaise, dry cough, and dyspnea for several weeks. Physical examination reveals tachypnea, tachycardia, and fever, with crackles on auscultation. On further questioning, the patient admits to IV drug abuse. The chest x-ray findings (top) prompt the clinician to order a chest CT study, from which is a representative section in the coronal plane is shown in the bottom figure.

What is the most likely diagnosis?

A. Pneumocystis pneumonia (PCP)
B. Pneumococcal pneumonia
C. Miliary tuberculosis (TB)
D. Cytomegalovirus (CMV) pneumonia
E. Pulmonary edema

Section III RADIOLOGY

Human Immunodeficiency Virus Pneumocystis Pneumonia (HIV PCP)

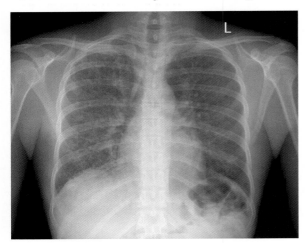

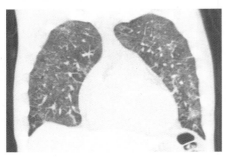

14. **The answer is A: Pneumocystis pneumonia (PCP).** The chest x-ray and chest CT show a diffuse ground-glass pattern throughout the lungs. The term *ground-glass* refers to the edge of a microscope slide that can be written on with pencil, and it means that although the area remains transparent, one cannot see detail through it. This pattern is characteristic of pneumocystis pneumonia, commonly known as *PCP*. The patient tested positive for HIV infection, likely acquired through the sharing of contaminated needles, and he is severely immunosuppressed. Sputum obtained during bronchoalveolar lavage was positive for PCP.

PCP is caused by *Pneumocystis jirovecii,* an endemic fungus that is harmless to immunocompetent individuals, but it is the most common cause of opportunistic infection in patients with HIV, typically occurring when CD4 counts fall below 200/μL. Although the organism is classified as a fungus, treatment is with antibiotics, trimethoprim-sulfamethoxazole, for 21 days. Despite antibiotic treatment, mortality rates range between 10% and 20%.

B. Pneumococcal pneumonia typically appears as a dense zone of lung consolidation, rather than a hazy ground-glass pattern. Pneumococcal pneumonia may occupy an entire lung lobe but is seldom a diffuse, bilateral process. Patients without a spleen are more susceptible to pneumococcal infection, because the organism is encapsulated and usually opsonized in the spleen. Patients with HIV, but still without clinical acquired immune deficiency syndrome (AIDS), have a higher incidence of pneumococcal infection than the general population.
C. Miliary TB characteristically appears as a diffuse micronodular pattern in the lungs, rather than a ground-glass pattern. The descriptive term *miliary* is derived from the appearance of tiny millet seeds which are used as bird feed. Miliary TB is a manifestation of TB bacteremia and can occur in both primary TB infection and in reactivation or secondary TB. TB has been considered an AIDS-defining illness in patients who are HIV positive.
D. CMV pneumonia is an opportunistic cytomegaloviral infection that occurs in immunosuppressed individuals, but it typically appears as a micronodular pattern, similar to miliary TB.
E. Pulmonary edema often appears as a ground-glass pattern on chest x-ray, but gravity dependence is characteristic, with relative sparing of the upper lungs. Patients in pulmonary edema should manifest other evidence of fluid overload or congestive heart failure, such as vascular congestion and pleural effusions.

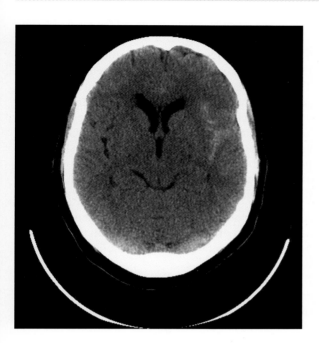

15. A 33-year-old woman presents to the emergency department with altered mental status and severe headache following a minor motor vehicle accident (MVA) in which she was the driver. The patient has no memory of the incident. The CT scan is above. The most likely explanation of the above finding is:

A. Posttraumatic subdural hemorrhage
B. Posttraumatic subarachnoid hemorrhage
C. Incidental calcification within the subarachnoid space
D. Subarachnoid hemorrhage (SAH) secondary to rupture of an aneurysm

Subarachnoid hemorrhage (SAH)

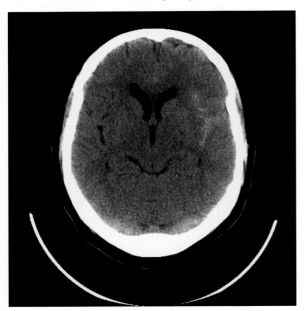

15. **The answer is D: Subarachnoid hemorrhage (SAH) secondary to rupture of an aneurysm.** The appearance is consistent with hemorrhage in the subarachnoid space (arrow). The distribution within the left sylvian fissure points to a ruptured aneurysm involving the left MCA region. CT angiography (CTA) or direct angiography should be performed urgently to identify the location of the aneurysm and treat it with either angiographically directed coiling or placement of a vascular clip.

A. Posttraumatic subdural hemorrhage is incorrect, as the location of the hemorrhage within the sylvian fissure is consistent with a subarachnoid, not subdural, location.
B. While SAH may be present following significant trauma, the MVA was described as minor. The distribution of blood in the sylvian fissure is more typical for an aneurysm rupture resulting in a loss of consciousness leading to her minor MVA.
C. Idiopathic calcification can occur. However, calcification is almost always related to a known previous insult, and the density is typically much greater than that seen on this image.

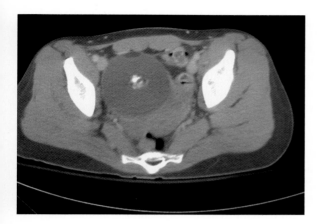

16. A 25-year-old woman is involved in a low-speed MVA and is taken to the emergency department. She is found to be stable, but is complaining of diffuse abdominal pain, and therefore a CT of the abdomen is obtained. Which of the following statements regarding the image provided is true?

A. There is active hemorrhage in the pelvis.
B. If left untreated, the salient abnormality can result in severe complications.
C. There is no malignant potential of the identified abnormality.
D. This abnormality has developed acutely.
E. This abnormality is found only in the pelvis.

Ovarian Teratoma

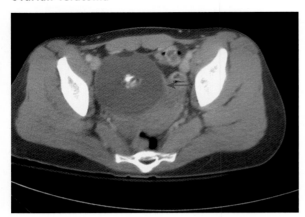

16. The answer is B: If left untreated, the significant pelvic abnormality can result in severe complications. The CT image provided demonstrates a round mass in the right hemipelvis, composed of central calcification, surrounding soft tissue, and less dense fat layering anteriorly (arrow). These findings are diagnostic of an ovarian teratoma. Despite being currently asymptomatic, this teratoma could potentially rupture, causing a chemical peritonitis and/or adhesions, act as a lead point in ovarian torsion, cause infertility due to mass effect on the fallopian tube or uterus, or rarely degenerate into a malignant teratoma, necessitating surgical resection with hope to preserve the ovary.

A mature ovarian teratoma is a benign neoplasm developing from at least two of the three primordial germ layers. Teratomas are the most common ovarian neoplasms in women younger than 20 years old. Ovarian teratomas can be bilateral in up to 15% of patients. Ultrasound, CT, and MRI are all potentially useful modalities in distinguishing teratomas from other ovarian neoplasms.

A. There is no evidence of hemorrhage on the image provided.
C. An ovarian teratoma may degenerate into a malignant teratoma, though it is rare.
D. This teratoma was likely present in this patient since birth, albeit smaller at that time.
E. In order of frequency, teratomas can arise from the sacrococcygeal region, gonads (ovarian and testicular), mediastinum, retroperitoneum, and intracranially (e.g., pineal gland).

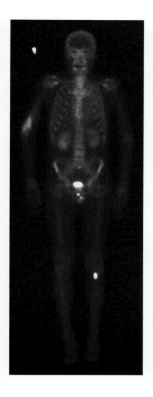
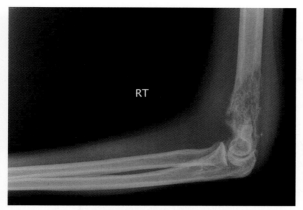
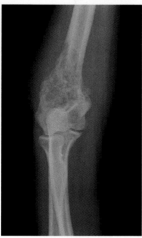
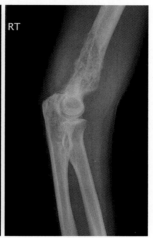

17. A 55-year-old woman with a history of breast cancer is found to have an elevated alkaline phosphatase on recent blood work and is sent for a bone scan. Based on the findings of the bone scan, radiographs are obtained. Based on the images provided, which of the following statements is true?

A. There is a solitary suspicious finding on the bone scan.
B. The radiographs are most compatible with an old healed fracture.
C. Bone scans are a sensitive modality for breast carcinoma metastases.
D. There is abnormal activity in the pelvis on the bone scan.
E. The findings on the bone scan and radiographs are disconcordant.

✎ *Notes*
_____

Lytic Bone Metastasis in Breast Cancer

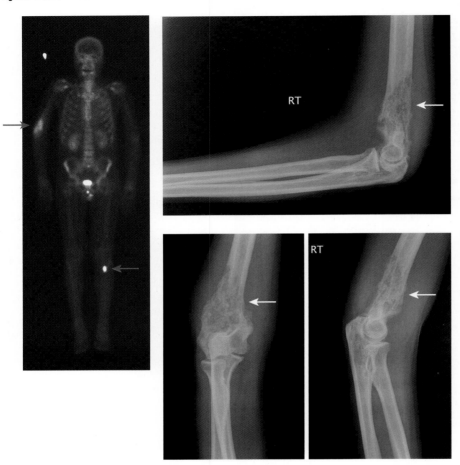

17. **The answer is C: Bone scans are a sensitive modality for breast carcinoma metastases.** The image from the bone scan above shows increased radiotracer uptake in the distal right humerus as well as in the proximal left tibia (red arrows). Given the history of breast cancer and an elevated alkaline phosphatase, these foci are very concerning for metastases. Bone scans are very sensitive for osseous metastases, particularly osteoblastic metastases, and are used as screening tools in patients with certain cancers, such as breast, prostate, and lung.

Breast cancer commonly metastasizes to bone, and can be either osteoblastic or osteolytic in nature. The 10-year survival rate of stage IV (metastatic) breast cancer is approximately 10%. In patients with suspicious findings on a bone scan screening for metastases, radiographs and, if necessary, MRI are appropriate imaging studies for further evaluation.

Bone scans are very useful in monitoring response to therapy in widespread metastatic disease to the bone.

A. As mentioned above, there are two suspicious lesions on the bone scan: on the distal right humerus and the proximal tibia. There is no abnormal activity elsewhere in the bones.
B. A pathologic fracture may be present on the lateral view, but is difficult to evaluate for with absent cortex. There is no healed fracture.
D. The bone scan radiotracer (Tc99m-MDP) is excreted via the kidneys; thus activity from urine within the bladder and urethra and on the perineum is normal.
E. The radiographs show a permeative, expansile, lytic process destroying the distal left humerus (white arrows), concordant with the bone scan findings and compatible with metastasis.

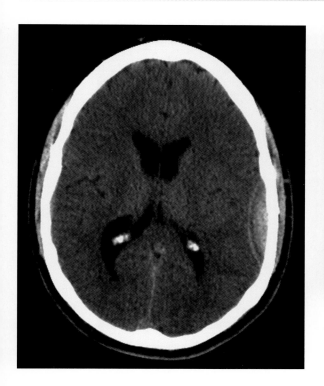
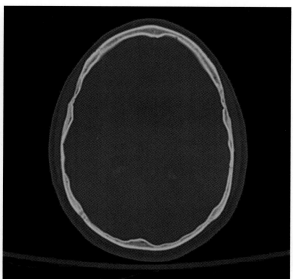

18. A 25-year-old man presents to the emergency department with a history of elbow to the head during a basketball game. He lost consciousness for a few minutes. Upon regaining consciousness, he was alert and oriented, complaining of a headache. By the time he arrived via ambulance, he complained of severe headache and was vomiting. A CT scan of the head was ordered and demonstrated the above findings. There is a hyperdense, biconvex collection in the left parietal region with a subtle, nondisplaced fracture of the left parietal bone.

The appearance above is most consistent with:

A. An acute subdural hematoma
B. A subacute to chronic subdural hematoma
C. An acute epidural hematoma
D. An acute epidural abscess

 Notes

Epidural Hematoma

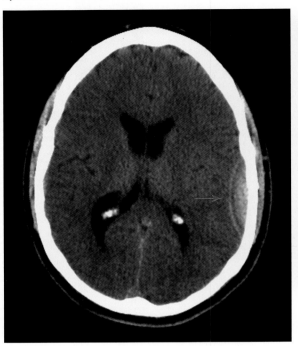
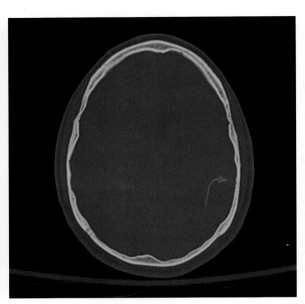

18. **The answer is C: An acute epidural hematoma.**
The history of trauma causing loss of consciousness with a lucid interval followed by a rapid deterioration in his clinical course is typical. Epidural hematoma (straight arrow) is usually caused by focal trauma to the temporoparietal region resulting in a fracture and tearing of the middle meningeal artery or one of its dural branches. On CT, the blood is hyperdense, lenticular, or biconvex in shape and does not cross suture lines. There is almost always a fracture associated with it, as in this case (curved arrow). It is a surgical emergency and, if untreated, is associated with a high mortality rate.

A. An acute subdural hematoma is frequently associated with trauma. The clinical presentation of a lucid interval is not typical. The source of the hematoma is venous rather than arterial, so there is usually a more indolent clinical course. On imaging, it frequently crosses suture lines as a crescentic hyperdense mass.

B. A subacute to chronic subdural hematoma would appear as an isodense to hypodense crescentic mass along the inner table of the calvarium. It is typically associated with either a remote trauma history or no known trauma history.

D. An acute epidural abscess would not present with this history. It is rare in the absence of intracranial surgery and typically has an insidious onset. On CT, an abscess should be hypodense rather than hyperdense.

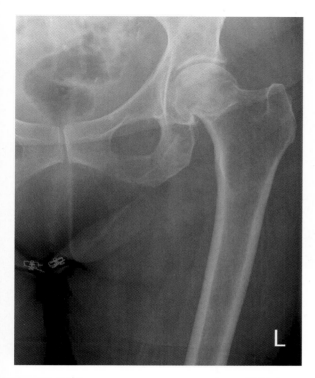

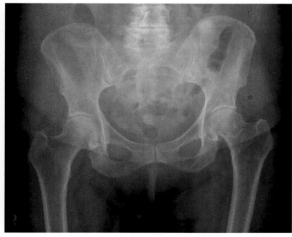

19. A 70-year-old woman suffers a fall at home and is brought to the emergency department by a neighbor. She is unable to walk and complains of pain in her left hip. Radiographs are obtained while she is in the waiting room. Which of the following statements is true?

A. This injury is the least common at this anatomic location.
B. This injury is often related to overuse.
C. There is a pathologic fracture.
D. There is an increased risk of avascular necrosis secondary to this injury.
E. This injury does not require surgery.

 Notes

Subcapital Femoral Neck Fracture

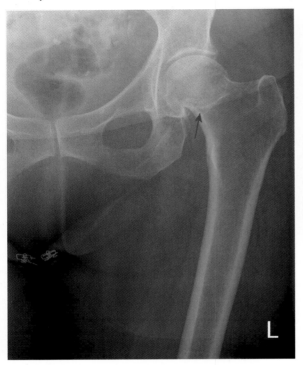
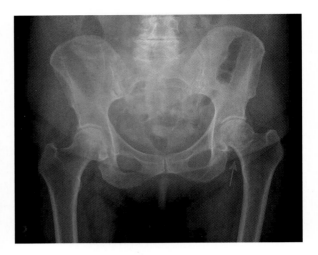

19. The answer is D: There is an increased risk of avascular necrosis secondary to this injury. This patient has suffered a displaced impacted subcapital fracture of the left femoral neck (red arrows). Femoral neck fractures are intracapsular with an increased risk of avascular necrosis from potential disruption of blood supply to the femoral head.

Femoral neck fractures are commonly sustained by elderly people, often related to seemingly mild falls. The propensity for the hip to flex and internally rotate when the femoral neck is fractured can obscure subtle fracture lines on radiographs. If a fracture is suspected and radiographs are negative, MR is the next most appropriate imaging study to perform. CT is much less sensitive for nondisplaced femoral neck fractures, usually because of the underlying osteoporotic bone.

Even with surgical fixation, the prognosis may be poor due to comorbidities such as venous thromboembolic disease and pneumonia.

A. Femoral neck fractures are described by location: subcapital, midcervical, and basicervical. The subcapital fracture is the most common. An intertrochanteric fracture is considered a proximal femoral fracture.
B. Insufficiency fractures commonly occur in the elderly, whereas overuse fractures commonly occur in young, extremely active people.
C. This fracture is simple (i.e., two fragments) with no evidence of an underlying pathologic process, such as metastasis.
E. The treatment for this fracture is internal fixation.

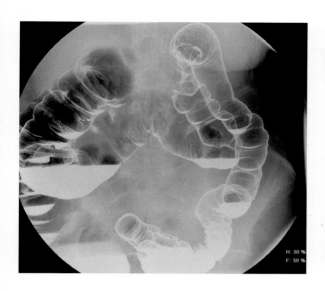
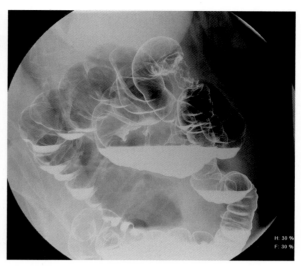
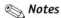

20. A 60-year-old woman presents to her primary care physician with weight loss and iron deficiency anemia. Fecal occult blood tests are positive. A double-contrast barium enema is performed for further evaluation. Which of the following statements is true regarding this disease?

A. Common risk factors include a high-fiber, low-fat, and animal protein diet, inflammatory bowel disease, and a positive family history.
B. This location is the most common site for this entity.
C. The treatment requires surgical resection, possibly with adjuvant chemotherapy.
D. These lesions are not associated with benign polyps.
E. This condition does not usually present with obstruction.

✎ *Notes*

Advanced Colon Carcinoma—Annular Constricting Lesion (i.e., Apple Core Lesion)

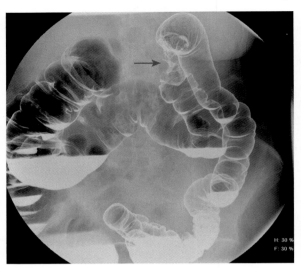 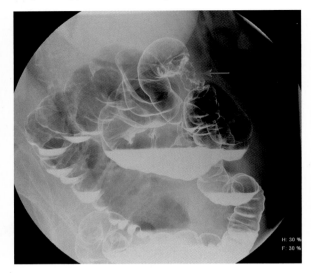

20. **The answer is C: The treatment requires surgical resection, possibly with adjuvant chemotherapy.** This vignette describes a classic presentation of colon cancer with the peak age at presentation of 50 to 70 years old and the most common presentations including weight loss, change in bowel habits, melena/hematochezia, and iron deficiency anemia. Colon cancer is the most common GI malignancy and the second most common cause of cancer deaths. Colon cancer can be identified on a barium enema as a sessile plaque, a pedunculated lesion, a large polypoid lesion, a semiannular or saddle-like lesion, an annular or apple core lesion, or wall thickening resembling a carpet-like lesion.

The spot radiographs above demonstrate circumferential narrowing in the distal transverse colon, with shelflike borders, resembling an apple core and representing an advanced annular constricting tumor (arrows). The barium enema has a 90%-95% detection rate for colon cancer, which is comparable with that of both colonoscopy and CT colonography. The advantage to the barium enema over colonoscopy in screening is the noninvasiveness. The advantage of colonoscopy in screening is the ability to remove polyps during the procedure. Both CT of the abdomen and pelvis and whole body positron emission tomography (PET) CT are useful modalities in initial staging of colon cancer, particularly in evaluating for lymph node and liver metastases.

A. Common risk factors include a low-fiber, high-fat (not low), and animal protein diet; inflammatory bowel disease; and a positive family history. Genetically based syndromes associated with an increased risk of colon cancer include familial adenomatous polyposis, Gardner syndrome, and hereditary nonpolyposis.
B. The sigmoid colon is the most common location, followed in order by the rectum, transverse, descending, and ascending colon, and cecum (the latter two being more common in advanced ages).
D. Most commonly, colon cancer is the result of malignant degeneration of a benign adenomatous polyp.
E. Fifty percent of colonic obstructions are caused by colon cancer, with other acute life-threatening complications being intussusception and perforation.

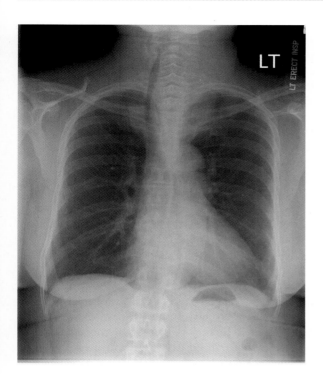

21. An asymptomatic, 50-year-old woman presents for preop testing prior to general anesthesia for knee replacement and has the chest x-ray shown above.

What is the most appropriate next step?
A. Barium swallow
B. CT of the neck and chest with contrast
C. CT of the neck and chest without contrast
D. Ultrasound of the neck
E. No additional imaging is needed before knee replacement surgery.

Section III RADIOLOGY

Thyroid Goiter

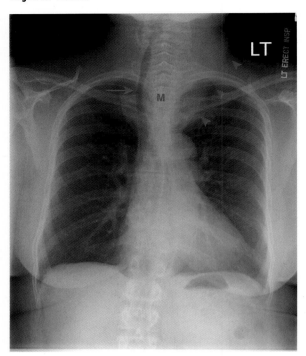

21. **The answer is C: CT of the neck and chest without contrast.** The next most appropriate step would be CT of the neck and chest without contrast to evaluate a large substernal goiter.

The chest x-ray shows a large mass (M) occupying the superior mediastinum and extending into the neck (arrowheads). The mass displaces the trachea to the right (arrow) and narrows the tracheal lumen along most of its length. The appearance is typical of a large substernal goiter. Further evaluation of the enlarged thyroid and its relationship to the trachea and great vessels is necessary prior to elective surgery under general anesthesia. Ideally the patient should be euthyroid at the time of surgery, so serum thyroid function tests and consultation with an endocrinologist are also indicated.

A. A barium swallow may be helpful in evaluation of the neck and esophagus in patients who are experiencing difficulty swallowing. However, a barium swallow would not provide detailed evaluation of the thyroid tissue or the extent of any encroachment on the trachea and great vessels.
B. CT imaging is ideal for evaluating the extent and the character of the thyroid mass, the patency of the trachea, and any encroachment on the great vessels in the superior mediastinum and the neck. However, the use of iodinated contrast is relatively contraindicated when evaluating the thyroid because the dye load saturates the thyroid gland with iodine. This would interfere with the uptake of radioactive I-131 for several weeks if there is a subsequent need for I-131 thyroid scanning or I-131 radiation therapy.
D. Ultrasound would provide insufficient imaging of this large, substernal goiter. Ultrasound of the neck is most appropriate for evaluation of a mildly enlarged gland that does not extend into the mediastinum or of a palpable thyroid nodule to determine if it is cystic or solid. Solid nodules may then be further evaluated with I-131 scanning. Benign adenomas take up iodine and appear "hot" on I-131 thyroid scans, whereas malignant nodules do not take up iodine and appear "cold."
E. Further imaging prior to elective surgery is necessary to evaluate any effect this very enlarged thyroid gland may have on the patient's airway and great vessels. If there were a need for emergency surgery, rather than elective surgery, an awake endoscopic intubation may be necessary to ensure a secure airway prior to induction of anesthesia.

There are many causes of thyroid goiter, and some of the more common etiologies are detailed below:

- The most common cause of goiter worldwide is dietary iodine deficiency. However, the common practice of iodine supplementation in salt makes this a less likely cause in the United States.
- Grave disease is a diffuse, benign enlargement of the thyroid gland. Grave disease is caused by autoimmune overstimulation of the thyroid that leads to thyroid hypertrophy, overproduction of thyroid hormone, and symptoms of hyperthyroidism.
- Hashimoto disease is caused by autoimmune damage to the thyroid that results in decreased thyroid hormone production and symptoms of hypothyroidism. Low serum thyroid hormone levels cause increased thyroid-stimulating hormone production by the pituitary which, in turn, stimulates thyroid growth.
- Multinodular goiters are caused by the presence of multiple, benign solid and cystic nodules throughout the gland that result in overall enlargement.
- Thyroiditis is an inflammatory condition of the thyroid that causes pain and generalized swelling.
- Several types of thyroid malignancy occur, but these typically manifest as a solitary, hard nodule rather than as diffuse glandular enlargement. A malignant nodule will appear as a solid nodule on ultrasound that is cold, or nonfunctioning, on I-131 thyroid scanning. CT imaging of malignant lesions may be helpful for evaluation of regional lymph nodes and staging.

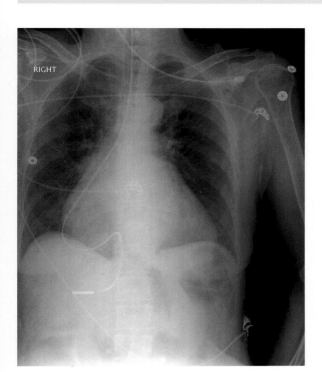

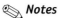

22. An 86-year-old woman is transferred for management of a recent stroke. She is breathing spontaneously but has difficulty swallowing. A portable chest x-ray is obtained following placement of a Dobhoff tube for enteric feeding.

Which of the following statements are true?
A. The Dobhoff tube is in satisfactory position in a patient with situs inversus.
B. The Dobhoff tube is in satisfactory position, after passing through a gastric pull-through and then below the diaphragm.
C. The Dobhoff tube is in satisfactory position, after passing through a large hiatal hernia and then below the diaphragm.
D. The Dobhoff tube is in the pleural space and should be removed.

Feeding Tube in Pleural Space with Pneumothorax

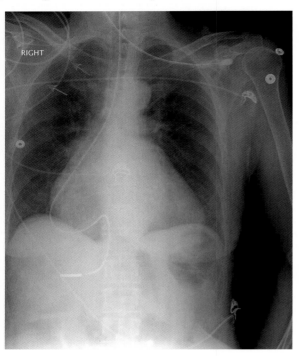

22. **The answer is D: The Dobhoff tube is in the pleural space and should be removed.**
The Dobhoff tube does not follow the expected anatomic course of the esophagus. Instead, it passes into the right main bronchus, then the right lower lobe bronchus, then perforates the right lung. The tip is deep in the right sulcus, in the pleural space, and it should be promptly removed.

As would be expected, there is also a right pneumothorax. The visceral pleural line (red arrows) is visible about 2 cm below the right upper ribs, with no lung markings beyond. Therefore, prompt chest tube placement is also indicated.

A. There is no situs inversus, as the gastric air bubble is visible just below the left diaphragm, and the liver occupies the right upper abdomen.

B, C. Sometimes a nasogastric (NG) tube or Dobhoff tube may follow a serpentine course if there is a dilated esophagus, a gastric pull-through following esophagectomy, a large hiatal hernia, or intrathoracic stomach. However, this patient shows no evidence of these entities. The gastric air bubble is in the expected location below the left diaphragm, and there are no clips in the chest or abdomen to suggest previous surgery. There is also no evidence of hiatal hernia, and the Dobhoff tube tip terminates outside the anatomic location of the stomach.

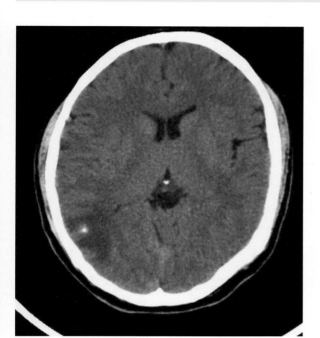

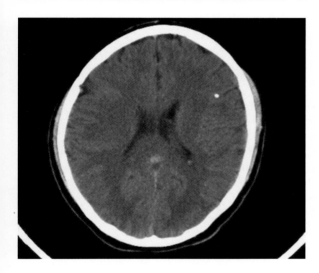

23. A 35-year-old Hispanic man presented to the emergency department with a history of worsening headache. While in the emergency department, the patient suffered a witnessed simple partial seizure. A CT scan of the head was obtained.

What is the most likely etiology for the above CT findings?

A. Congenital
B. Infectious
C. Inflammatory
D. Metabolic
E. Toxic

Neurocysticercosis

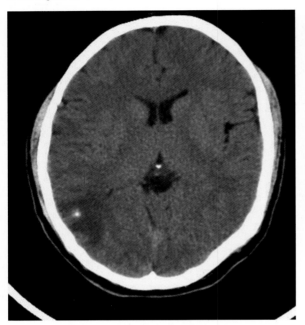
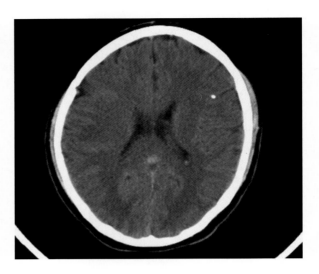

23. **The answer is B: Infectious.** The finding of focal calcifications (arrowheads) in both the left frontal lobe (image on right) and right parietal lobe (image on left) is a classic presentation for neurocysticercosis. There is a surrounding hypodensity (straight arrows) and mass effect involving the calcification in the right parietal lobe, representing edema. This calcification with accompanying edema represents a more acute stage of disease demonstrating an active host response while the left frontal calcification represents a later, inactive stage. Neurocysticercosis is common in developing countries and is being seen more often in developed countries like the United States with the continued immigration from Central and South America.

The presentation is nonspecific, and seizure is not uncommon.

A. If it were congenital, one would expect to find migrational anomalies with gray matter heterotopia, which is not seen in these images.
C. The image on the left demonstrates edema, which is expected in an inflammatory condition; however, the second image demonstrates a single calcification without any inflammatory changes.
D. Most metabolic processes affect the brain more diffusely and symmetrically.
E. As with metabolic processes, there is typically a more diffuse and symmetric appearance to the abnormality.

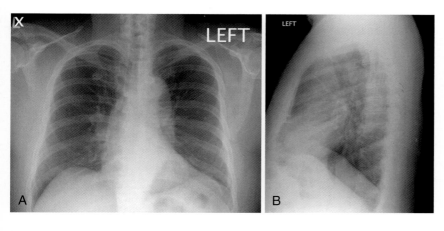

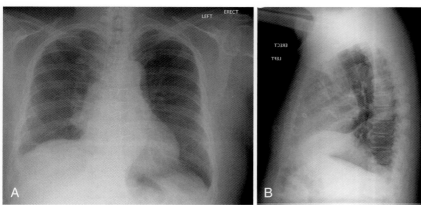

24. A 77-year-old man has a normal preoperative chest x-ray (top, A and B) prior to coronary arterial bypass graft. His hospital course proceeds uneventfully, and he is discharged for outpatient rehabilitation. At his 6-week postoperative checkup, he reports persistent dyspnea without chest pain or palpitations, especially with exercise or when lying down. The ECG shows no changes, and the lungs sound clear on exam. A follow-up chest x-ray (bottom, A and B) is obtained for further evaluation.

What is the most likely diagnosis?

A. Congestive heart failure
B. Dressler syndrome
C. Subpulmonic effusion
D. Right lower lung collapse
E. Right phrenic nerve palsy

Paralyzed Diaphragm

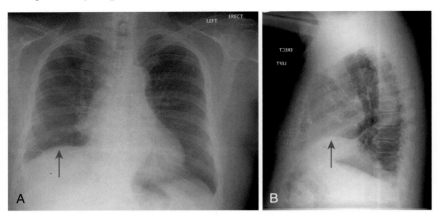

24. **The answer is E: Right phrenic nerve palsy.**
The phrenic nerves derive from the C3, C4, and C5 cervical roots bilaterally and pass caudally through the neck and mediastinum to innervate the two leaves of the diaphragm. Phrenic nerve palsy can be caused by inadvertent surgical interruption of the nerve during mediastinal dissection, as in this case. Other possible etiologies include trauma or, most commonly, malignant invasion.

The most common symptom is dyspnea which is exacerbated with exercise and recumbent positioning. The chest x-ray shows elevation of the affected diaphragm (arrows). Diagnosis can be confirmed by fluoroscopic observation of respiratory motion. The affected diaphragm does not descend like the opposite, normal diaphragm on inspiration. A "sniff test" maneuver, in which the patient abruptly sniffs, causes sharp inspiration of the normal diaphragm, which increases abdominal pressure that in turn causes paradoxical elevation of the paralyzed diaphragm.

A. Patients with congestive heart failure may present with dyspnea. However, the chest x-ray would show evidence of pulmonary edema and pleural effusions.
B. Dressler syndrome is a self-limited autoimmune phenomenon that occurs several weeks after myocardial exposure from bypass surgery or myocardial infarction. Left-sided chest pain relieved by aspirin is the characteristic symptom. The chest x-ray characteristically shows a small left-sided pleural effusion.
C. This patient has no pleural fluid. Pleural effusions usually pool in the costophrenic angles with a characteristic meniscus shape. Occasionally fluid collects below the lung, elevating the lung base, and this is known as a *subpulmonic effusion*. Detection may be difficult on the PA chest x-ray, although the diaphragm contour is subtly abnormal, and a meniscus is usually visible posteriorly on the lateral view. A decubitus view allows the fluid to pool along the lateral chest, confirming diagnosis.
D. This patient's right lower lung remains inflated even though the right diaphragm is elevated from phrenic nerve palsy. In cases of right lower lung collapse, the airless lobe appears as a focal increased density at the medial right lung base on the PA view and at the posterior base on the lateral view. The right diaphragm edge is typically effaced on the PA view because there is no right lower lobe air to outline it.

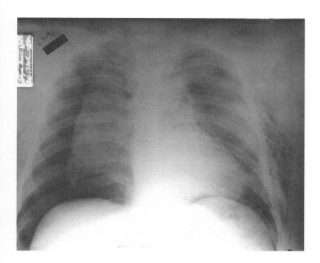

25. A 33-year-old healthy man is in the operating room being prepared for inguinal hernia repair. Intubation is unexpectedly difficult, and after a traumatic intubation, the patient is noted to be hypoxic. A stat portable chest x-ray is obtained.

What is the diagnosis?

A. Hyperaeration
B. Left pneumothorax
C. Right pneumothorax
D. Right tension pneumothorax
E. Bilateral pneumothorax

Deep Sulcus Pneumothorax

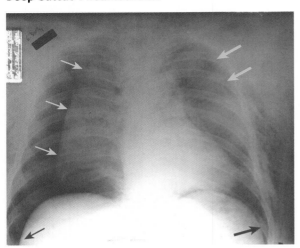

25. **The answer is E: Bilateral pneumothorax.** Traumatic intubation may lead to tear of the trachea, piriform sinus, or esophagus, and pneumothorax and/or pneumomediastinum may result. Once the patient is stabilized, further evaluation of the integrity of the airway and esophagus should proceed. CT scanning, Gastrografin studies, and endoscopic evaluation may all be helpful.

A, B, C, D. The thorax is hyperinflated, not from pulmonary hyperaeration, but from bilateral pneumothoraces.

The portable chest x-ray shows complete collapse of the dense, airless right lung, which has the appearance of a spinnaker sail (narrow yellow arrows). A large right pneumothorax surrounds the collapsed lung, and it is obvious that there are no lung markings in the periphery of the chest. Perhaps less obvious is the telltale "deep sulcus sign" (narrow red arrow) which appears as hyperlucency at the right lung base, with an unusually deep costophrenic angle, because in the supine position a pneumothorax may sometimes be most visible at the lung base, rather than at the apex.

The mediastinum is shifted toward the left, indicating that the right pneumothorax is indeed under tension, with imminent risk of cardiovascular compromise. Therefore, prompt chest tube placement to relieve the pneumothorax is imperative.

On closer inspection, the x-ray also shows evidence of a moderate-sized left pneumothorax (wide yellow arrows). The edge of the left lung is displaced about 2 cm from the ribs, and there is a deep sulcus sign at the left base, as well (wide red arrow).

Observation of the additional left-sided pneumothorax reinforces the importance of doing a complete and organized search of the image, even if an obvious abnormality is present. Failure to observe additional abnormalities is sometimes called *happy eye syndrome,* which describes the tendency to quit looking once the first observation provides "satisfaction of search."

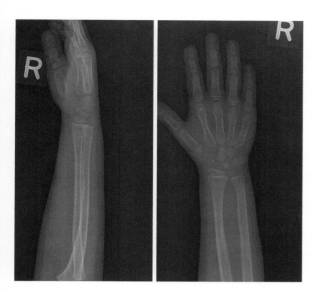

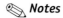

26. Which of the following best describes the injury?

  A. Toddler fracture
  B. Greenstick fracture
  C. Stress fracture
  D. Buckle/torus fracture
  E. Plastic fracture

Buckle/Torus Fracture of Distal Radius and Ulna

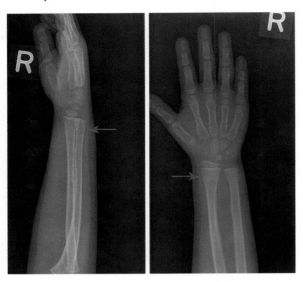

26. **The answer is D: Buckle/torus fracture.** The radiographs show buckle fractures of the distal radial and ulnar metaphyses (red arrows). The word *buckle* denotes the "buckling" of the cortex. The cortex can buckle in or out, and when buckled out, it appears as a protuberance along the otherwise smooth cortex, often in a circumferential fashion, as seen in the case above. The word *torus* denotes a circular protuberance, which has been attributed to an elevated intact periosteum due to subperiosteal hemorrhage.

A buckle, or torus, fracture is one of many fractures that can commonly be seen in skeletally immature patients in whom the increased elasticity of the bone (relative to an adult) results in deformation rather than a break. The "ball bearing rule" implies that a ball bearing would jump at the site of the fracture if rolling down the cortex. These fractures tend to heal completely with immobilization (casting) and only rarely develop a subperiosteal cortical defect. Buckle fractures are usually due to axial loading, sometimes with an angular component, and when in the distal radius, especially the metaphysis, are often the manifestation of the skeletally immature falling on an out-stretched hand.

The buckle fracture is often included in the category of incomplete fractures (not involving the entire cortex); other such fractures include plastic, greenstick, stress, and toddler.

A. A toddler fracture is a fracture occurring in the legs or feet of those children who are just beginning to ambulate without other trauma. A common toddler fracture involves the distal tibia, often in a spiral configuration.
B. In a greenstick fracture, the cortex is usually disrupted or bowed on one side of the bone, the side that experienced the causative tension, resembling a broken green twig.
C. In an early stress fracture, the bone subjected to repetitive stress may appear normal on radiographs, or it may have barely visible hairline fractures.
E. In a plastic fracture, the bone bends without a cortical deformity.

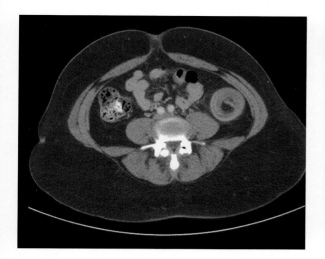

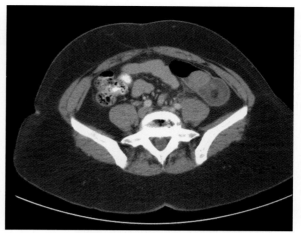

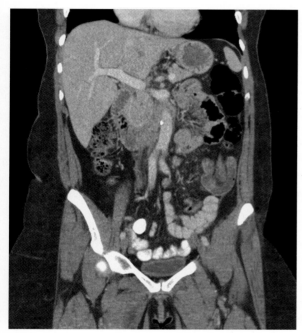

27. A 55-year-old woman with no significant past medical history presents to the emergency department with severe, intermittent, diffuse, abdominal pain, worsening over the course of a few days. Physical examination is pertinent for abdominal tenderness in the left lower quadrant. There is no blood per rectum. Vital signs are stable, and laboratory values are normal. A CT of the abdomen is obtained. Based on the images provided, which of the following statements is true?

 Notes

A. The salient abnormality is within the right lower quadrant.
B. A predisposing condition responsible for an acute process is identified.
C. There is a small bowel obstruction.
D. Nonsurgical management is preferred.
E. The emergency department physician should immediately consult the urology service.

Intussusception—Colocolonic with Lead Point Mass

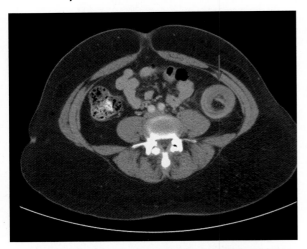

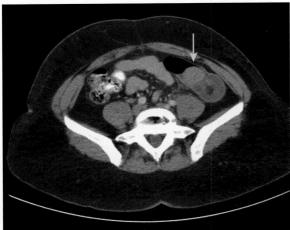

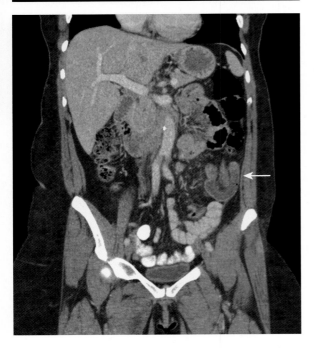

27. The answer is B: A predisposing condition responsible for an acute process is identified. The findings on the images provided are pathognomonic for intussusception, colocolonic in this case. On the first axial image provided, there is a classic "target sign" in the left lower quadrant, with a bowel within bowel appearance peripherally, more central mesenteric fat, and a mesenteric vessel as the bull's eye (red arrow). On the second axial image, a rounded soft tissue mass is seen in the more distal descending colon (yellow arrow), which is acting as a lead point, pulling with it a segment of more proximal descending colon and its mesentery.

Intussusception occurs when a proximal segment of bowel telescopes into a more distal segment, often pulling the mesentery with it (white arrow). Complications of intussusception include obstruction and compromise of the vascular supply to the bowel that results in bowel ischemia, perforation, and sepsis. Long segment intussusception is relatively rare in adults and is almost always due to a lead point mass or Meckel diverticulum. Intussusception is more common in children than adults, and is most commonly ileocolic and idiopathic. In such cases, the initial preferred treatment is pneumatic reduction with an air enema.

A. The salient abnormality is within the *left* lower quadrant.
C. There is no evidence of a small bowel obstruction, with the visualized small bowel loops normal in caliber, without wall thickening, and containing intraluminal contrast.
D. In adults, long segment, nontransient intussusception, particularly with a lead point identified, usually requires surgery, especially if there is evidence of vascular compromise. The mass in this case was found at surgery to be a colon polyp. Short segment intussusception, especially in the small bowel, tends to be a transient phenomenon, not requiring long-term follow-up or intervention.
E. There is no genitourinary surgical issue necessitating a urology consult.

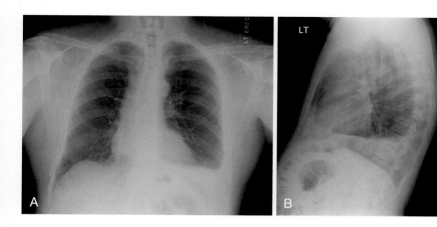

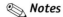

28. A 58-year-old construction worker undergoing routine physical examination for life insurance evaluation is found to have decreased breath sounds at the left lung base, and a chest x-ray is ordered for further evaluation.

Based on the x-ray interpretation, which of the following diagnoses must be considered?

A. Metastatic lung cancer
B. TB
C. Mesothelioma
D. All of the above

Mesothelioma

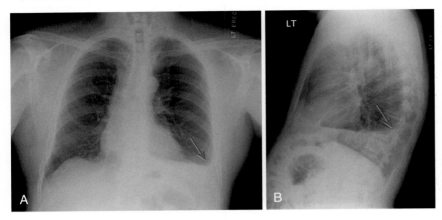

28. **The answer is D: All of the above.** The chest x-ray shows a small left pleural effusion (red arrows) with no visible lung abnormality, and all three diagnoses, metastatic lung cancer, TB, and mesothelioma, must be considered as possible causes.

This patient had a primary mesothelioma, and a follow-up chest x-ray 6 months later showed a significantly larger left effusion. PET CT (below) done for further evaluation at that time showed the large effusion (e) and a metabolically active, irregular soft-tissue mass along the diaphragmatic surface (white arrow), consistent with pleural malignancy.

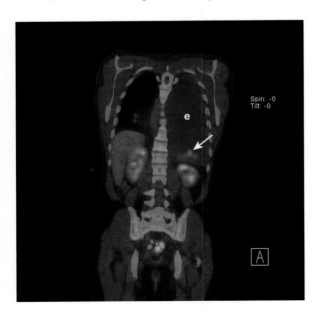

Mesothelioma is a primary pleural malignancy with poor prognosis. Pericardial and peritoneal mesothelioma also occur but with less frequency. Occupational exposure to asbestos is an almost uniform underlying risk factor, although patients seldom have true asbestosis, which is an asbestos-related interstitial lung disease.

The onset of malignancy is typically decades following initial exposure to crocidolite-type asbestos fibers. Clinical symptoms of mesothelioma include dyspnea, cough, chest discomfort, weight loss, and anemia. Characteristic chest x-ray findings include effusion, pleural thickening, and pleural-based masses or nodularity. Although some patients undergo thoracotomy for surgical excision, prognosis remains poor, and palliative treatment is appropriate.

The differential diagnosis of unilateral left effusion is lengthy and includes both benign and malignant, as well as acute and chronic, etiologies. Malignant effusions may be caused by primary mesothelioma or by pleural metastasis from many possible primary cancers, including lung, breast, GI, ovarian, lymphoma, and many others. Infectious causes of unilateral effusion include primary TB and bacterial empyema, which typically produces a loculated effusion. Certain autoimmune diseases such as rheumatoid arthritis and lupus may produce small left effusion. Dressler syndrome is a self-limited, autoimmune process that occurs after myocardial infarction or after cardiac surgery and presents as a small left effusion associated with left chest pain. In patients with history of trauma or surgery, a unilateral hemorrhagic or chylous effusion may occur. Abdominal disease processes such as pancreatitis, subdiaphragmatic abscess, or ascites may also give rise to unilateral effusion. Cirrhosis typically produces a larger, right-sided effusion. Other common causes of effusion, such as congestive heart failure, are most often bilateral and usually show underlying pulmonary edema.

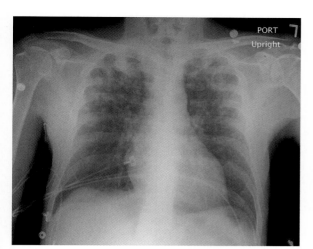

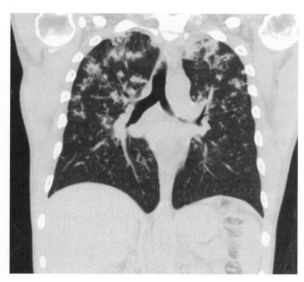

29. An HIV-positive, 54-year-old man presents to the emergency department complaining of cough and malaise. On further questioning, he admits to IV drug abuse, and he has experienced intermittent sweats and weight loss over the last 4 months. A chest x-ray (top) and chest CT (bottom) were obtained.

What is the most likely diagnosis?

A. Septic emboli
B. Pneumococcal pneumonia
C. PCP
D. Metastasis
E. TB

TB in HIV

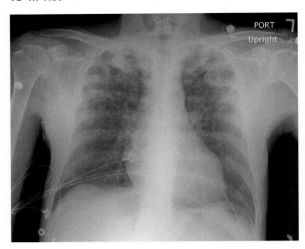

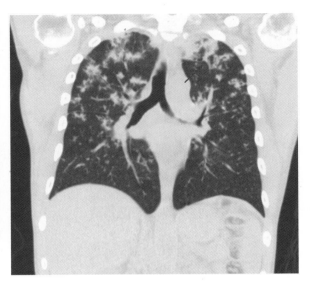

29. **The answer is E: TB.** The patient has characteristic symptoms and x-ray findings of active TB, and prompt respiratory precautions are indicated. Clinical symptoms of active TB can be myriad and include cough, malaise, night sweats with intermittent fevers, and weight loss. As in this patient, x-rays typically show patchy, heterogeneous consolidations, predominantly in the better-aerated upper lobe zones. There may be cavitation (arrows), sometimes with air-fluid levels. Other possible findings include pleural effusion, pericardial effusion, and hilar or mediastinal adenopathy, especially in children. Chest CT commonly demonstrates evidence of endobronchial spread of infection with infectious material distributed in the distal airways.

The causative bacterium is *Mycoplasma tuberculum,* which is endemic in underdeveloped countries and often seen among recent immigrants as well as impoverished individuals. TB has been considered an AIDS-defining illness in HIV-positive patients, who are particularly susceptible. The infection is spread through inhaled microdroplets produced during coughing as well as during talking. Therefore, the patient's mouth and nose should be covered until antibiotic treatment renders sputum samples free of

acid-fast bacilli, and all close contacts of the patient should be screened for TB.

A. Septic emboli may be suspected in patients with fever and history of IV drug abuse. They appear as faint, rounded nodules on chest x-ray, sometimes with evidence of central necrosis. Chest CT shows multiple cavitary and solid nodules showered throughout the peripheral lungs, with no upper lobe predominance.
B. Pneumococcal pneumonia occurs with greater frequency in HIV-positive patients than in the general population. However, the typical chest x-ray and CT findings would show dense lobar consolidation with air bronchograms, which represent lucent airways branching through the zone of infection.
C. PCP is an opportunistic infection commonly seen among HIV-positive patients, particularly when the CD4 count falls below 200. The typical chest x-ray and CT findings are of a vague, ground-glass, infiltrative pattern with scattered air bronchograms. The distribution tends to be diffuse but heterogeneous.
D. Pulmonary metastases may have a variety of patterns, including lung nodules, cavitary lesions, and infiltrative interstitial patterns. However, they tend to be widely distributed without upper lobe predominance.

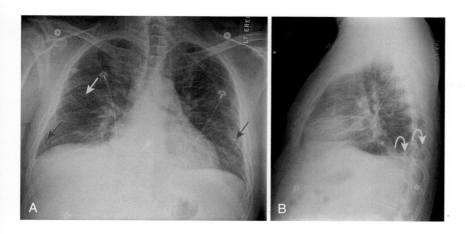

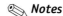

30. A 53-year-old man presents to the emergency department with chest pain and shortness of breath. The ECG shows elevated ST segments. A chest x-ray is obtained which shows diffuse coarsening of the interstitial markings, with Kerley A lines (straight yellow arrow), Kerley B lines (red arrows), and small bilateral pleural effusions (curved yellow arrows).

What is the significance of the Kerley A and B lines on the chest x-ray?

A. The patient has pulmonary interstitial edema.
B. The patient is developing acute respiratory distress syndrome (ARDS).
C. The patient has metastatic lung cancer.
D. The patient has asbestosis.
E. The patient has *Mycoplasma* pneumonia.

Acute Myocardial Infarction with Kerley Lines

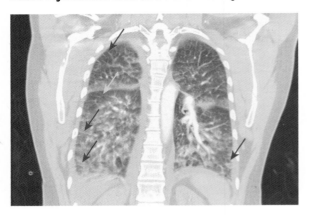

30. **The answer is A: The patient has pulmonary interstitial edema.** Dr. Peter Kerley, a radiologist from Ireland, described A, B, and C lines on radiographs as representing distended pulmonary lymphatics in patients with fluid overload or congestive heart failure. Kerley A lines (yellow arrow) are long lines radiating from the hila to the periphery, and they represent lymphatic distention in the intralobular septae. Kerley B lines (red arrows) are short, peripheral linear densities that represent distended lymphatics in the interlobular septae. Kerley C lines appear on the chest x-ray as a fine network of crisscrossing lines and represent superimposed A and B lines (not apparent on image shown).

The chest x-ray shows a central and bibasilar ground-glass pattern associated with small effusions and Kerley A and B lines. In the clinical setting of chest pain, dyspnea, and ECG changes, the chest x-ray findings are diagnostic of pulmonary edema. A chest CT (shown above), obtained for other reasons, confirms the findings.

B. In patients with ARDS, the pulmonary capillaries lining the alveoli are damaged, and fluid seeping into the alveolar air spaces creates a diffuse ground-glass pattern. However, since there is no fluid overload, and no distention of the lymphatics, no Kerley lines and no pleural effusions should be present.

C. Lung cancer metastasis in the chest may manifest as multiple pulmonary nodules; as pleural metastasis with malignant effusion; as hilar and mediastinal adenopathy, which may obstruct central vessels; and as lymphangitic spread of tumor. When there is central venous obstruction from adenopathy or when the lymphatic channels are invaded, there will be lymphatic obstruction and distention, with appearance of unilateral or bilateral Kerley lines. Although lymphangitic carcinomatosis is in the differential diagnosis when Kerley lines are observed, this patient's clinical scenario is highly characteristic of an acute myocardial infarction with pulmonary edema.

D. Asbestosis is a pneumoconiosis caused by inhalation of asbestos dust, which may incite pulmonary interstitial fibrosis. However, the increased interstitial lung markings in patients with asbestosis tend to be coarser in texture with more distortion of the lung architecture. Calcified pleural plaques often accompany the interstitial abnormalities in patients with asbestosis.

E. *Mycoplasma* pneumonia is a common community-acquired pneumonia that typically demonstrates lung infiltrates and interstitial prominence. Patients with *Mycoplasma* have clinical evidence of upper respiratory tract infection, but no clinical or chest x-ray evidence of fluid overload or vascular congestion.

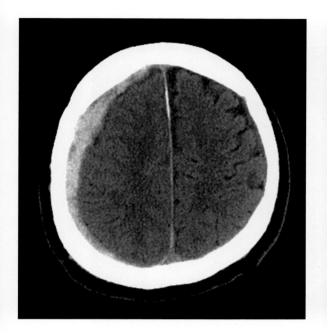
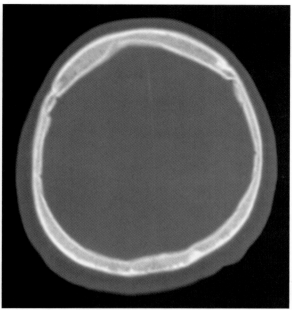

31. An 82-year-old man presents to the emergency department with a complaint of persistent headache for the past week following a fall from standing. Cranial nerve and mental status exams are normal. The CT scan is shown above.

The finding above most likely represents:

A. Subarachnoid hemorrhage
B. Subdural hemorrhage
C. Epidural hemorrhage
D. Epidural abscess

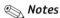 *Notes*

Subdural Hemorrhage

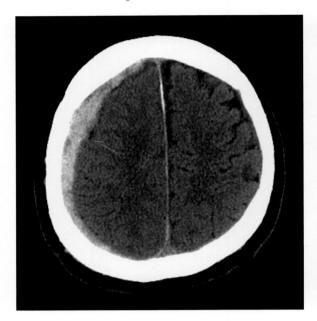
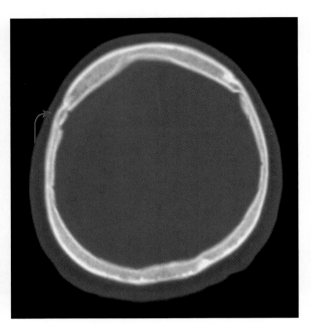

31. **The answer is B: Subdural hemorrhage.** In the elderly patient, because of the cerebral volume loss and stretching of the cortical veins, minor trauma such as a fall from standing may cause these veins to tear, with blood accumulating in the subdural space. The appearance of a hyperdense crescentic collection (straight arrow) crossing suture lines (curved arrow) is classic for an acute subdural hematoma.

A. Subarachnoid hemorrhage may occur as a result of trauma. Its distribution is typically within the sulci, and it does not displace brain parenchyma.

C. Epidural hemorrhage may displace brain parenchyma but typically is associated with severe trauma resulting in fracture of the calvara with resultant tearing of an epidural artery. It is typically a lenticular-shaped collection that does not cross suture lines. Due to its arterial supply, it can rapidly expand, resulting in herniation and death. It is a surgical emergency.

D. Epidural abscess is typically a hypodense collection. The patient usually presents with other symptoms supporting infection and altered mental status.

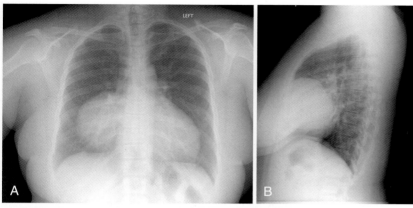

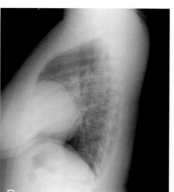

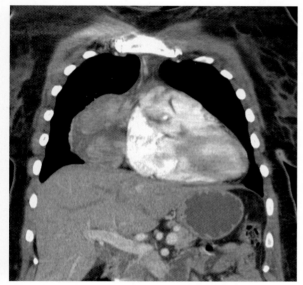

32. A 38-year-old, asymptomatic woman presents for a preoperative chest x-ray (top) prior to bunionectomy. The chest x-ray findings prompt further examination with chest CT (bottom).

What is the most likely diagnosis?

A. Pericardial cyst
B. Lymphoma
C. Thymoma
D. Teratoma
E. Diaphragmatic hernia

Thymoma

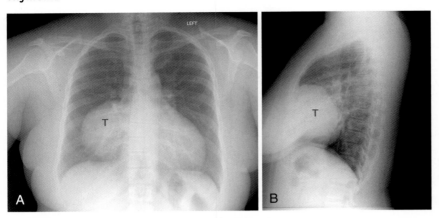

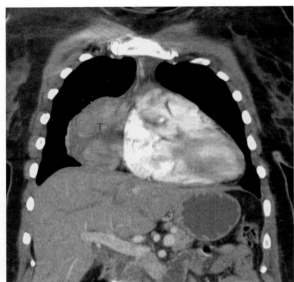

32. **The correct answer is C: Thymoma.** There is a large soft tissue mass (T) in the right anterior mediastinum, with a solid, heterogeneous appearance most suggestive of thymoma. Incidentally found thymomas are not uncommon, although symptoms such as chest discomfort may be present. Of patients with thymoma, 30%-50% have associated symptoms of myasthenia gravis, but only 15%-20% of patients with myasthenia

have an underlying thymic tumor. The general differential diagnosis of anterior mediastinal masses includes lymphoma, other causes of adenopathy, thymic lesions, germ cell tumors such as teratoma, and thyroid masses such as substernal goiter.

A. Pericardial cysts are fluid-filled lesions with a thin mesothelial lining, usually along the right heart border. This lesion is clearly solid with no fluid component.
B. Lymphoma may present as an asymmetric mediastinal mass and is statistically more common than thymoma. However, a more typical appearance would be a homogeneous, solid mat of adenopathy in the prevascular space of the superior mediastinum. Many other causes of bulky adenopathy, such as sarcoid or metastatic disease, can also occur in the anterior mediastinum but are less likely in an asymptomatic patient.
D. Teratomas and other germ cell tumors include all three germ cell layers and typically feature fatty components that are obviously radiolucent on CT studies. Teratomas often show calcifications and sometimes partially formed teeth or bones.
E. This patient's diaphragm is intact with no evidence of rupture or herniation. Herniation is usually left-sided but may occur on the right and may contain liver, colon, and/or omentum.

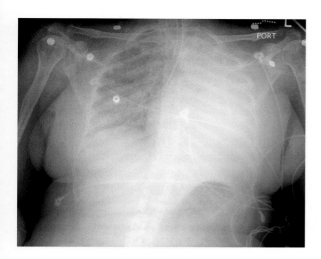

33. A 41-year-old woman in the intensive care unit with congestive heart failure shows persistent evidence of oxygen desaturation despite intubation for respiratory distress.

After interpreting her portable chest x-ray, what is the next appropriate action?

A. NG tube placement
B. Chest tube placement
C. Administration of IV furosemide
D. Endotracheal tube (ET) tube adjustment
E. A left lateral decubitus chest x-ray

Lung Collapse

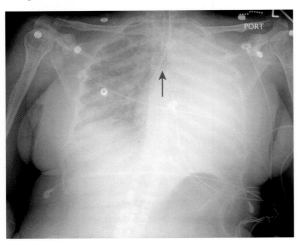

33. **The answer is D: Endotracheal (ET) tube adjustment.**
The chest x-ray shows pulmonary edema in the right
lung and complete opacification, or white-out, of the
left hemithorax. The causes of an opacified hemithorax
include complete lung collapse, large pleural effusion,
dense lobar pneumonia, and prior pneumonectomy.
A clue to the presence of lobar collapse may be
noticeable shift of the mediastinum toward the affected
side, caused by volume loss in the airless lung. In large
effusions, the mediastinum usually remains midline.
Lung consolidation from lobar pneumonia is seldom
this densely opaque, and lucent branching airways,
known as *air bronchograms,* are typically visible in
zones of dense lung consolidation. Patients with prior

pneumonectomy show typical postsurgical changes
such as metallic clips and sometimes surgical rib
defects.

In this case, the ET tube is below the carina in
the right mainstem bronchus, and only the right
lung is being ventilated. The left lung has absorbed
all available oxygen from the airways and has
collapsed, producing complete opacification of the
left hemithorax. If the ET tube is withdrawn 5 cm, it
will be above the carina (arrow), and the left lung will
reexpand.

A. There is evidence of moderate gastric distention
in the left upper abdomen, likely from air swallowing
during intubation. This places the patient at some
risk of aspiration, but placement of an NG tube
is secondary, relative to the imperative of ET tube
adjustment.
B. A chest tube would be indicated to drain a large
pleural effusion, but this patient has a collapsed lung
and no effusion.
C. The right lung shows evidence of pulmonary edema,
and the patient may benefit from IV furosemide.
However, ET adjustment is the first priority.
E. A left lateral decubitus x-ray is helpful in
determining the presence of free-flowing left
pleural effusion. However, a decubitus view offers
no clarification when effusions are so large as to
produce complete opacification of the hemithorax.
Furthermore, the cause of this patient's white-out is
lung collapse, not effusion.

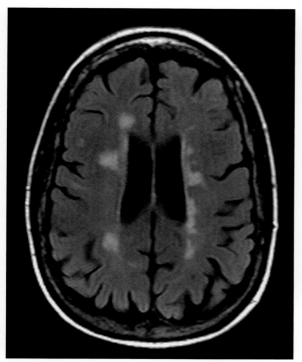

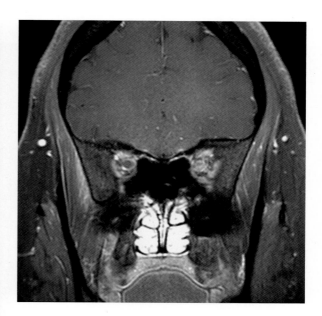

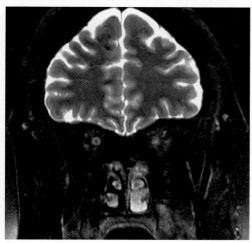

34. A 38-year-old woman presents to her physician's office with a complaint of acute onset of blurry vision and pain in her left eye. Her medical history is otherwise unremarkable. The MRI demonstrated enhancement of the left intraorbital segment of the optic nerve on coronal postcontrast T1 imaging corresponding to optic nerve edema demonstrated on the coronal T2 imaging. Axial fluid attenuated inversion recovery (FLAIR) imaging of the brain demonstrated multiple hyperintense lesions predominantly periventricular in location.

Her blurry vision is most likely related to:

A. Ischemic optic neuropathy
B. Orbital pseudotumor
C. Optic neuritis
D. Orbital cellulitis

 Notes

Optic Neuritis Multiple Sclerosis

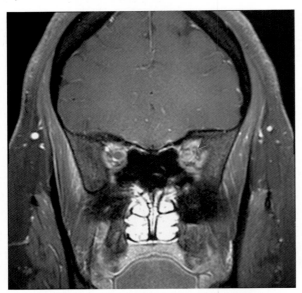

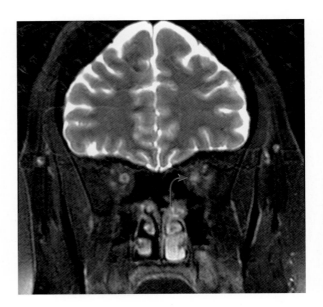

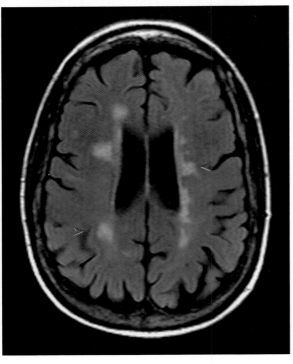

34. **The answer is C: Optic neuritis.** The clinical symptoms described are a typical presentation of the disease. Optic neuritis is an inflammatory demyelinization that is associated with an increased risk of developing multiple sclerosis. There is enhancement of the optic nerve (straight arrow), with optic nerve edema (curved arrow). The most significant predictor for the subsequent development of multiple sclerosis is the presence of white matter lesions on FLAIR imaging of the brain (arrowheads). Their perpendicular orientation to the lateral ventricles is typical for multiple sclerosis.

A. Ischemic optic neuropathy secondary to atherosclerotic disease typically presents with painless vision loss and is typically in an older age group. The imaging characteristics are relatively nonspecific.
B. Orbital pseudotumor typically presents with the acute onset of pain, swelling, proptosis, and decreased vision. In the absence of other signs suggesting infection, the diagnosis is frequently made clinically, and the patient is put on steroids.
D. Orbital cellulitis presents with proptosis and ophthalmoplegia. It is frequently accompanied by other signs and symptoms of infection including fever, pain, decreased vision, and chemosis. It is usually apparent clinically.

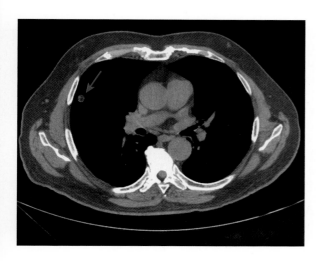

35. A 63-year-old healthy man with no smoking history has a lung nodule incidentally discovered on a preoperative chest x-ray for knee arthroscopy. Chest CT confirms a 9-mm solitary pulmonary nodule (arrow) in the right middle lobe with no other abnormalities.

What is the next appropriate step?

A. Purified protein derivative (PPD) placement
B. PET scanning
C. CT guided lung biopsy
D. Follow up CT scan in 1 year
E. No further evaluation is needed

Solitary Lung Nodule

35. **The answer is E: No further evaluation is needed.**
The CT scan shows that the solitary lung nodule contains lucent fat deposits characteristic of a benign hamartoma. Therefore, no treatment or follow-up imaging is needed.

Hamartomas are the most common benign neoplasms of the lung and are the third most common cause of a solitary lung nodule. They are more common in men than in women and typically present as an incidental chest x-ray finding in middle-aged patients. Pathologically they represent benign neoplasms that contain a variety of lung tissues including fat, benign epithelial cells, and often cartilage, which may exhibit calcification. Therefore, the CT appearance is often diagnostic, especially if the lesion contains fat or popcorn-type calcification.

The differential diagnosis of a nonspecific-appearing, solitary pulmonary nodule is extensive, including both benign and malignant etiologies, although, fortunately, most are benign. The most common etiologies are active or dormant infection and primary or metastatic malignancies.

Indications for further evaluation of a nonspecific solitary nodule depend on the patient's risk factors for malignancy and on the size and appearance of the nodule. Factors which increase the patient's risk of malignancy include smoking history, exposure to asbestos or radon, past history of malignancy, advanced age, and a larger-sized or spiculated nodule. Factors which increase the likelihood of benign etiology include lack of smoking history, positive PPD, young age, small nodule, and the presence of fat or calcification in the nodule. The presence of calcification is readily detectable with CT and vastly improves the likelihood of benign etiology such as a granuloma from TB or histoplasmosis.

Table 3-1 summarizes general recommendations and shows that one may conclude, for example, that a 25-year-old nonsmoker with a 3-mm nodule needs no further evaluation; however, a 65-year-old heavy smoker with a 9-mm nodule may want to consider biopsy, or certainly further evaluation with PET CT.

A. PPD placement is not necessary in this case, because the lung nodule is obviously a benign hamartoma. However, PPD status would be helpful in weighing risk factors for a nonspecific, noncalcified nodule.
B. PET CT is not needed for evaluation of this benign lesion. However, PET CT may be helpful in determining the likelihood of malignancy of an ambiguous nodule that measures at least 1 cm.
C. Biopsy is not indicated for this benign lesion. However, biopsy of a 9-mm, nonspecific nodule may be considered, especially in a high-risk patient.
D. No follow-up is indicated in this case. However, a 9-mm, nonspecific nodule without calcification or fat would require close follow-up if biopsy were not performed, even in a low-risk patient. Multiple follow-up scans would be needed to document short-term stability, beginning at 3 months, and long-term stability, ending at 2 years. A one-third increase in diameter, from 9 mm to 12 mm, would represent a volume double, and if this occurred over a 6-month period, it would represent a suspicious pattern of growth that would prompt biopsy.

Table 3-1

Nodule Size	Low-Risk Patient	High-Risk Patient
Nodule ≤ 4 mm	No follow-up required	Follow-up CT @ 12 months; if stable, stop
Nodule = 4–6 mm	Follow-up CT @ 12 months; if stable, stop	Follow-up CT @ 6–12 months; if stable, then CT @ 18–24 months
Nodule > 6–8 mm	Follow-up CT @ 6–12 months; if stable, then CT @ 18–24 months	Follow-up CT @ 3–6 months; if stable, then 9–12 months; if stable, then 24 months
Nodule > 8 mm	Follow-up CT @ 3, 9, 24 months—dynamic CT w/contrast, PET, and/or biopsy	Follow-up CT @ 3, 9, 24 months—dynamic CT w/contrast, PET, and/or biopsy

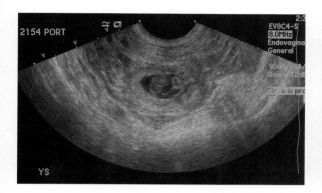
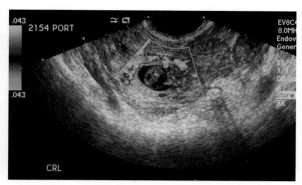
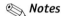

36. A 20-year-old woman presents to the emergency department with crampy lower abdominal pain and some vaginal bleeding. Her last menstrual period was approximately 2 months ago; however, her cycles are irregular. A serum beta HCG level is 50,000 mIU/mL. Which of the following statements is true regarding the images of the right adnexa above obtained from a transvaginal ultrasound with color Doppler analysis?

A. A gestational sac is present, and it is within the uterus.
B. While a gestational sac is present, there is no embryo or yolk sac identified.
C. Color Doppler analysis demonstrates no significant abnormality in the right adnexa.
D. A right ovary appears separate from the gestational sac.
E. The approximate age of this fetus is 18 weeks.

✎ Notes

Ectopic Pregnancy

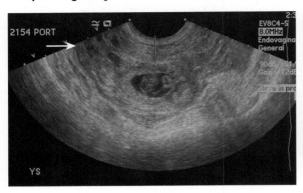 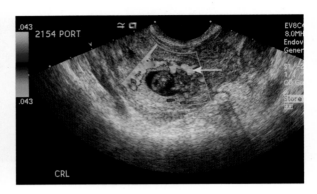

36. **The answer is D: A right ovary appears separate from the gestational sac.** The images of the right adnexa obtained from a transvaginal ultrasound with color Doppler analysis demonstrate an ectopic pregnancy in the fimbrial/infundibular region of the right fallopian tube. On the first provided image (above left), the right ovary, containing multiple hypoechoic subcentimeter follicles, is seen to the right and slightly anterior to the right ovary (white arrow), and abuts the gestational sac (red arrow) at an acute angle with a thin amount of echogenic adnexal tissue intervening.

An ectopic pregnancy is defined as any gestation occurring outside of the uterus or within the cornua of the uterus, and can lead to high morbidity and mortality if diagnosis is delayed. Ninety-five percent of all ectopic pregnancies are tubal. Essential sonographic findings for diagnosing an ectopic pregnancy in women with a positive beta HCG include no intrauterine pregnancy and an adnexal/tubal mass. If there is no intrauterine pregnancy and an adnexal mass is not identified, ectopic pregnancy cannot be excluded, and the patient requires close follow-up with serial beta HCG levels and, if needed, repeat ultrasounds. Treatment options for ectopic pregnancy include medical management (e.g., with oral methotrexate), surgical management with salpingectomy, or ultrasound guided percutaneous injection of the gestational sac with potassium chloride.

A. While images of the uterus are not provided to exclude a concurrent intrauterine pregnancy (so-called heterotopic pregnancy), this gestational sac is certainly not within the uterus.

B, E. No measurements are provided to accurately date the embryo; however, the crown-rump length of the embryo is slightly more than 10 mm based on the scale provided on the side of the image (each dot representing a sonometer), and there is still a yolk sac, making this pregnancy clearly within the first trimester.

C. On color Doppler (above right), there is a semicircle of increased blood flow surrounding the gestational sac, which is compatible with the so-called ring of fire sign attributed to an ectopic pregnancy (yellow arrow). Care must be taken to prove that the ectopic pregnancy is separate from the ovary. An ovarian ectopic pregnancy is extremely rare; however, a corpus luteum within the ovary can also have a ring of fire appearance, leading to false positives. If there were further question as to whether the mass/gestational sac was ovarian in origin, the ultrasound probe could be used to apply pressure to the ovary. If the ovary moves independently from the gestational sac, then they are truly separate structures.

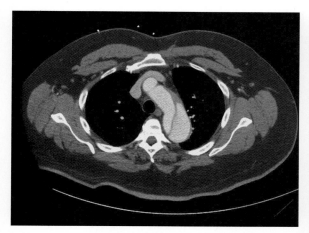

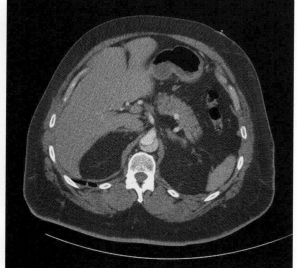

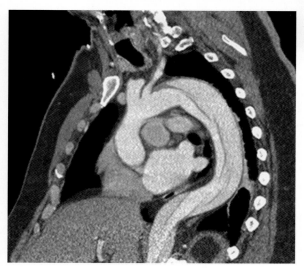

37. A 60-year-old man with hypertension presents to the emergency department with tearing back pain. A CT-angiography (CTA) of the thorax is obtained. Classically, how is this disease process managed?

A. Watchful waiting
B. Endovascular graft placement
C. Medical management (i.e., lower blood pressure)
D. Aortic bypass
E. Aortic valve replacement

 Notes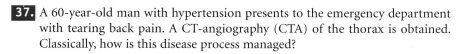

Aortic Dissection—Type B

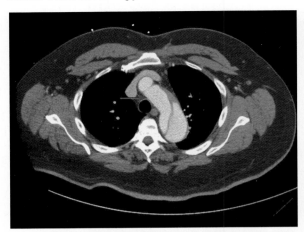

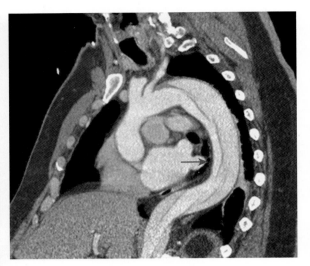

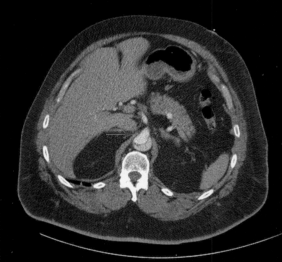

37. The answer is C: Medical management (i.e., lower blood pressure). This patient is presenting with an acute thoracic aortic dissection, type B. Aortic dissection occurs when an intimal disruption results in a subintimal hematoma that can expand to compress the true aortic lumen (red arrows). The false lumen can propagate in either a proximal or distal direction with potential to obstruct aortic branch vessels.

Under the preferred classification system, the Stanford system, there are two types of dissections: type A originates in the ascending thoracic aorta, and

type B originates distal to the left subclavian artery. Type B dissections are classically treated with medical management if major branch vessels, such as the superior mesenteric artery, communicate with the true aortic lumen, as in this case. The mortality rate of those with type B dissections treated with medical management is 10%.

Aortic dissection is a life-threatening emergency with a very high mortality rate, necessitating rapid diagnosis with CTA in suspected patients. On CTA, an intimal flap with a contrast-enhancing intramural hematoma (i.e., false lumen) is diagnostic. In patients who have contraindications to IV contrast, MR angiography and transesophageal echocardiography are alternative imaging modalities. In patients with chest pain, ischemic heart disease is at least 1000 times more common than aortic dissection.

A. Untreated dissections have a mortality rate of approximately 1%-2% per hour for the first 48 hours, making watchful waiting an inappropriate response.
B, D. Type A dissections are typically treated with endovascular graft placement, with a mortality rate of 30%.
E. Type A dissections can compromise the origins of the coronary arteries and the aortic valve, which may necessitate valve replacement.

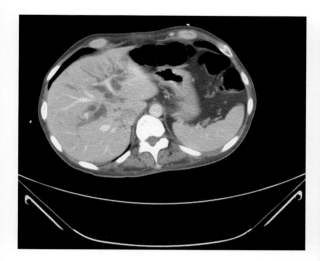
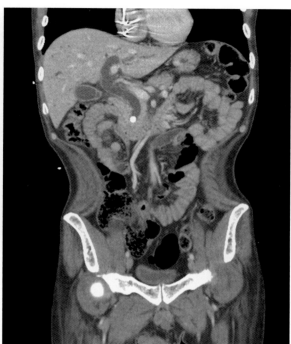

38. A 50-year-old man with no past medical history presents to the emergency department with new yellowing of his skin and eyes. He denies any abdominal pain. Aside from elevated bilirubin, his serum chemistries are normal. Based on the images from the contrast-enhanced CT of the abdomen above, what is the diagnosis?

A. Sclerosing cholangitis
B. Cholangiocarcinoma
C. Adenocarcinoma of the pancreatic head
D. Obstructive choledocholithiasis
E. Portal vein thrombosis

 Notes

Obstructive Jaundice—Choledocholithiasis

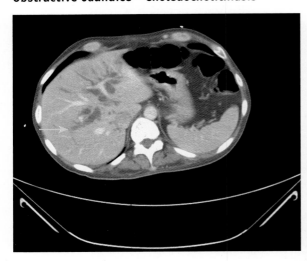
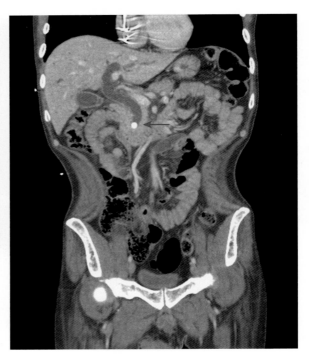

38. **The answer is D: Obstructive choledocholithiasis.**
This patient is presenting with painless jaundice.
The classic etiology of painless jaundice in a middle-
aged individual is pancreatic carcinoma, and this CT
of the abdomen was obtained to evaluate for such.
However, it was fortunate for this patient that the
CT clearly demonstrated an obstructing calculus in
the distal common bile duct (red arrow), within the
pancreatic head, with resulting marked extrahepatic
and intrahepatic biliary ductal dilatation. This
presentation is somewhat atypical for obstructive
choledocholithiasis, because patients often experience
pain. The dilatation of the common bile duct leading
to the common hepatic duct and left hepatic duct
is seen well on the coronal image. The axial image
demonstrates the marked dilatation of central
intrahepatic biliary radicals (a yellow arrow identifies
one such radical in the right hepatic lobe).

Causes of common bile duct obstruction include
choledocholithiasis, pancreatic or ampullary
neoplasms, benign stricture, and parasite infection.
The density of gallstones is variable on CT, with
calculi ranging from less dense than water, isodense
to water (therefore invisible), or calcified as in
this case. MR cholangiopancreatography (MRCP),
ultrasound, and hepatobiliary scintigraphy, often
prove more sensitive imaging modalities in suspected
choledocholithiasis. In an acute presentation of
obstructive jaundice, CT of the abdomen with
contrast is an appropriate first-line imaging
modality to evaluate for neoplastic and potentially
infectious or autoimmune causes. Endoscopic
retrograde cholangiopancreatography (ERCP) with
sphincterotomy and calculus retrieval is a preferred
initial therapy in obstructive choledocholithiasis.

A. While sclerosing cholangitis is a cause of
obstructive biliary dilatation, the most common
finding on CT is scattered dilated intrahepatic bile
ducts that do not clearly communicate with the biliary
system, and, again, there is a more clearly identifiable
etiology on the provided images.
B. Likewise, there is no intraluminal or intrahepatic
mass on these images to support a diagnosis of
cholangiocarcinoma.
C. On the provided coronal image, no pancreatic head
mass is seen, and furthermore, a clear cause of the
biliary dilatation is identified.
E. The visualized portions of the portal vein system,
seen adjacent to the dilated intrahepatic biliary ducts
and common bile duct on the coronal image, are
enhancing normally.

Images for Question 39 on page 254.

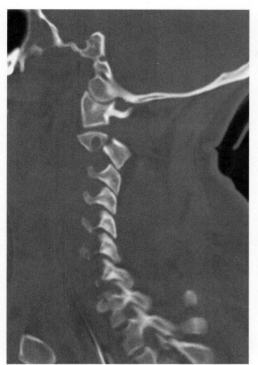
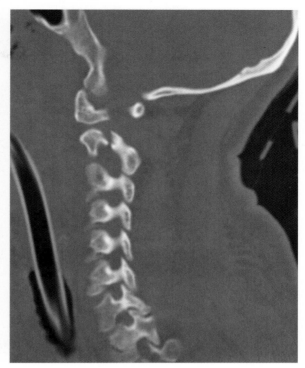
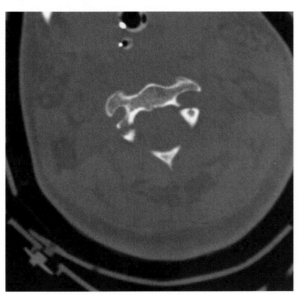

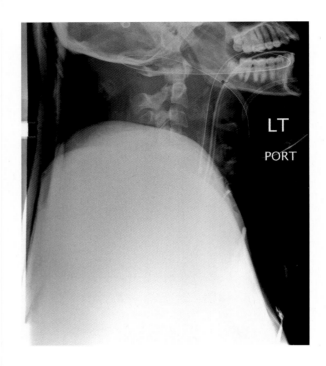

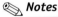 **Notes**

---

39. Following a high-speed MVA, an unrestrained 47-year-old woman passenger is transported by air to the nearest trauma center. The patient required intubation at the accident scene, but responds to commands and is found to be neurologically intact on examination. A CT of the cervical spine is performed. Based on the findings, the patient is taken for a stat MRI and then taken for surgery. An intraoperative lateral radiograph of the cervical spine is obtained (shown above). Based on the images provided, which of the following statements is true?

A. This type of cervical spine fracture is considered stable.
B. Spinal cord edema and/or hemorrhage will definitely be seen on the MRI.
C. Cervical MR angiography should be performed at the same time as the MRI.
D. This type of injury has been named a *Jefferson fracture.*
E. The mechanism of injury producing this fracture classically is hyperflexion.

Hangman's Fracture (explanation on p. 256)

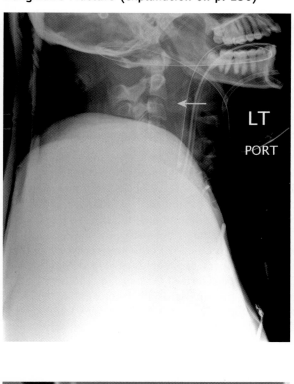

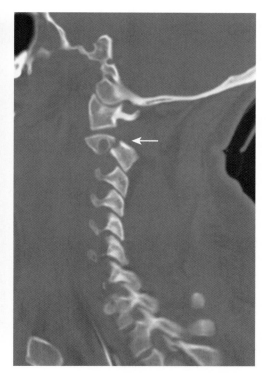

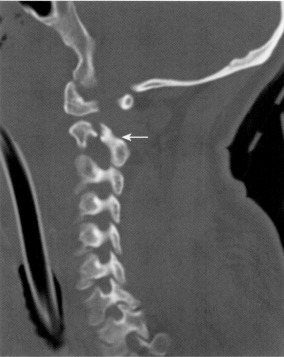

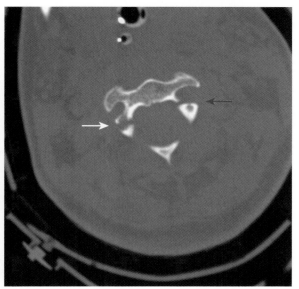

39. **The answer is C: Cervical MR angiography should be performed at the same time as the MRI.** The patient has suffered traumatic spondylolisthesis of the axis (TSA), commonly known as the *hangman's fracture*. The sagittal CT images above show bilateral traumatic spondylolysis at C2, or fractures through the pars interarticularis on both sides of the posterior neural arch of C2 (white arrows). On the lateral radiograph, although subtle, there is trace anterolisthesis, or anterior translation of C2 on C3 (yellow arrow). This subluxation would likely be exaggerated if neck flexion were allowed. The axial CT image shows that the fracture on the left extends into the foramen transversarium (red arrow), through which the left vertebral artery travels. Vertebral artery injury is a relatively common potential complication, especially when the fracture extends into the foramen transversarium, as seen with this case. Cervical MR angiography is a useful additional sequence to be performed with the expected conventional MRI of the cervical spine to evaluate for vertebral artery injury.

The term *hangman's fracture* is commonly used, though anachronistic, to describe TSA. This injury was originally named based on historical accounts of such fractures occurring during hangings, when the knot of the noose was placed under the chin and violently forced upwards under the weight of the victim. Today, of those still hanged for capital punishment, only a minority is found to have C2 arch fractures, and MVAs and falls account for a majority of such injury patterns. In high velocity trauma victims, when cervical spine injury is suspected, CT is a more appropriate first-line imaging study than radiographs. MRI is extremely useful in evaluating for nonosseous injury, such as traumatic disc herniation, epidural hematoma, and ligamentous damage.

A. While the fracture is considered unstable and requires surgical fixation, neurologic deficits occur in only about 25% of cases, likely due to the relative capaciousness of the spinal canal at C2 and the potential for autodecompression from the fracture. **B.** Cord edema and/or hemorrhage would be a less likely finding on the MRI of the cervical spine of this neurologically intact patient for the reasons cited in A. **D.** This has been termed the *hangman's fracture*. A Jefferson fracture classically denotes a four-part break through the anterior and posterior arches of the C1 ring. **E.** The mechanism of this fracture is usually forced hyperextension with axial loading, and is often the result of the chin striking the dashboard in a motor vehicle crash.

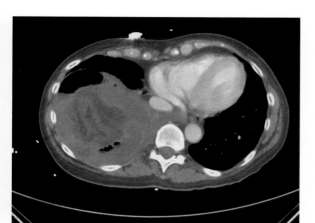

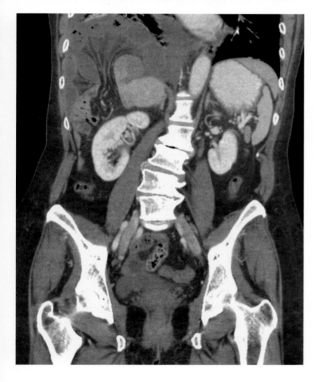

40. A 50-year-old woman is brought to the emergency department with severe abdominal pain that has worsened over the course of about a week. She is also dyspneic. Her past medical history is significant for injuries sustained in an MVA 1 year ago. Pertinent physical exam findings include decreased breath sounds in the right lung base, and abdominal guarding and rebound tenderness. She is tachycardic with a borderline low blood pressure. Her serum lactate is elevated. Which of the following statements is true regarding the findings on the select images provided from a CT of the abdomen?

A. Findings are most consistent with complicated pneumonia in the right lung base.
B. The visualized bowel is normal.
C. This acute process is likely the sequela of remote trauma.
D. The patient has a good prognosis with surgical management.
E. The right hemidiaphragm is intact.

Diaphragmatic Rupture with Strangulated Intrathoracic Herniated Bowel

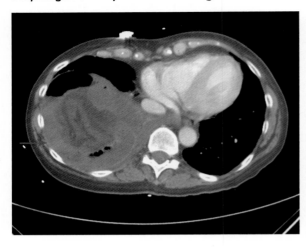

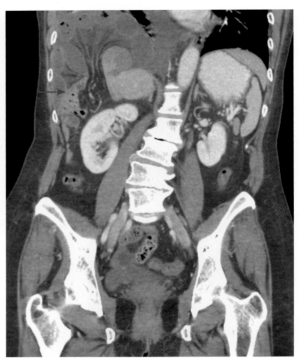

40. **The answer is C: This acute process is likely the sequela of remote trauma.** The CT images above demonstrate herniation of small bowel and mesentery into the thorax through a traumatic diaphragmatic rupture (red arrows). In the acute setting of trauma, diaphragmatic rupture is often difficult to diagnose and may remain clinically silent for a long period of time until complications arise, such as in this case.

Strangulated herniated bowel is a life-threatening emergency requiring immediate surgery. Diaphragmatic rupture can result both from blunt abdominal trauma, due to increased intraabdominal pressure, and from penetrating trauma, from direct laceration from a projectile or stabbing weapon. CT is the best initial study in a patient with an acute abdomen, especially if diaphragmatic rupture is within the differential diagnosis. Nontraumatic diaphragmatic hernias include Bochdalek hernia (posterolateral), Morgagni hernia (anteromedial), and hiatal hernias.

A. While there is likely compressive atelectasis in the right lung base from the herniated mass, there is no consolidative process in the visualized lungs.
B. The herniated bowel is dilated with fluid, and the bowel wall is thickened and hypoenhancing, indicating obstruction and strangulation or vascular compromise.
D. The mortality in cases of strangulated GI diaphragmatic hernia is reported as up to 60%.
E. Again, the right hemidiaphragm is obviously not intact.

Images for Question 41 on page 260.

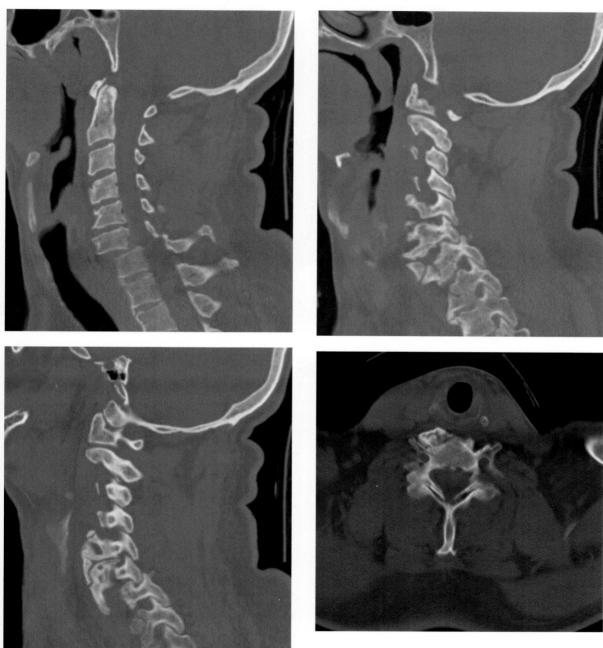

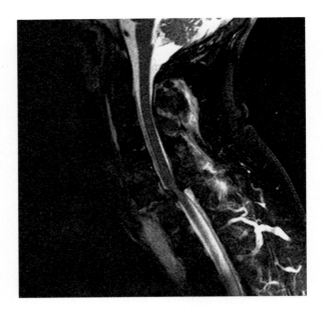

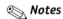 *Notes*

41. A 21-year-old man is brought to the nearest trauma center after a diving accident from a large height. A CT of the cervical spine is performed (see images on p. 259), followed immediately by an MRI of the cervical spine (shown above). Based on the images provided, which of the following statements is true?

A. The axial CT image shows an additional osseous abnormality.
B. This injury is considered stable.
C. There is no soft tissue injury.
D. There is no damage to the cervical spinal cord.
E. There is high incidence of tetraplegia associated with these injuries.

Bilateral Interfacetal Dislocation—Jumped Facets

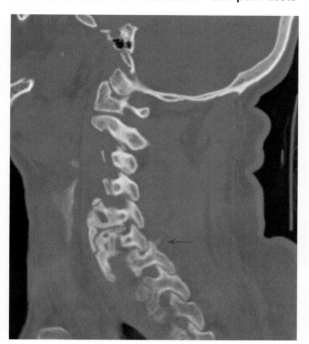
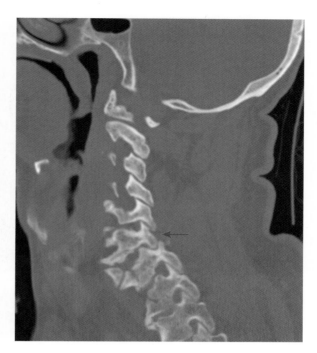

41. **The answer is E: There is high incidence of tetraplegia associated with these injuries.** The CT images above demonstrate bilateral interfacetal dislocation with jumped facets. The sagittal CT images through the facet joints shows both of the superior articulating masses dislocated anterior to the inferior articulating masses (red arrows), with loss of the normal shinglelike alignment. Additionally, on the MR images, as would be expected, the spinal canal is severely narrowed, with impingement of the cervical cord and cord edema at the level of dislocation (yellow arrow). Given the evidence of cervical cord injury, tetraplegia is quite likely, as is common in such injuries.

Bilateral interfacetal dislocation is a severe injury of the mid to lower cervical spine caused by extreme hyperflexion. In hyperflexion injuries, facets can be widened, perched (inferior tip of superior facet in contact with superior tip of inferior facet), or jumped. Other hyperflexion type injuries include hyperflexion sprain, simple wedge compression fracture, and flexion tear drop fracture. Evaluation with both CT and MRI of the spine is essential to determine the extent of osseous and soft tissue injury, respectively.

A. The axial CT image demonstrates the same finding, and illustrates the so-called reverse hamburger sign (white arrows), where the facets, representing the halves of a hamburger bun, appear flipped and upside down in relation to each other.

B, C. The sagittal CT image through the midportion of the vertebral bodies shows greater than 50%

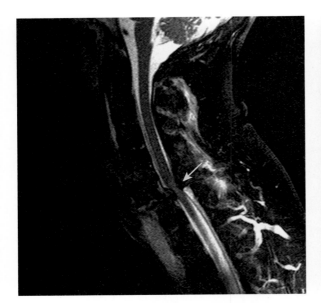

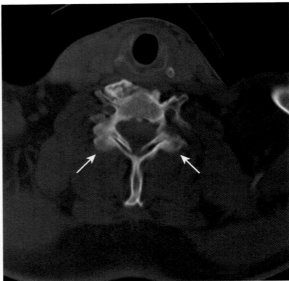

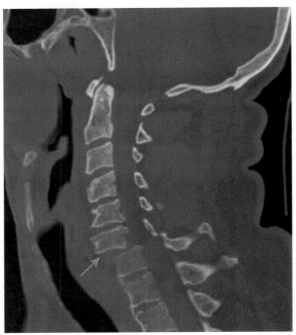

subluxation of the C6 vertebral body anteriorly on the C7 vertebral body (green arrow). In order for the cervical vertebra to translate anteriorly, there must be disruption of nearly all of the supporting ligamentous structures of the spine at that level, including the anterior longitudinal ligament, the intervertebral disc, the posterior longitudinal ligament, the ligamentum flavum, and the interspinous ligaments, making it an inherently unstable injury. Edema can be seen within a majority of the aforementioned ligamentous structures and in the prevertebral soft tissues on the MR images provided.

D. There is cervical cord injury as evidenced by the impingement of the cervical cord and cord edema.

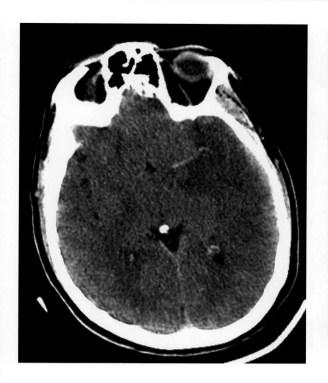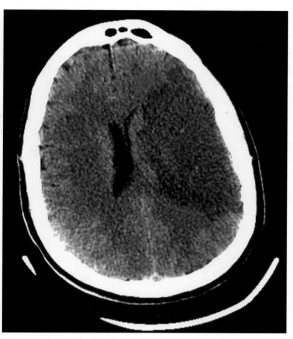

42. A 63-year-old man presents with a history of acute onset of left hemiparesis and dysarthria 12 hours before his arrival to the emergency department. A CT scan was ordered. The best next step in his management is:

A. Oral administration of 325 mg aspirin
B. Emergent administration of intraarterial recombinant tissue plasminogen activator (rtPA)
C. Emergent CT perfusion study to assess for the amount of tissue at risk
D. Emergent angiographic intervention with thrombectomy

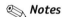 **Notes**

MCA Infarct

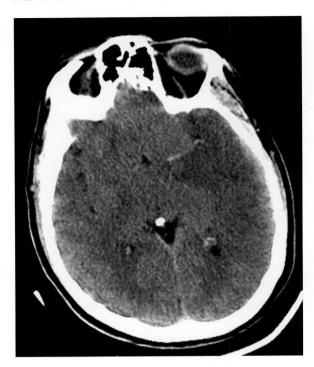 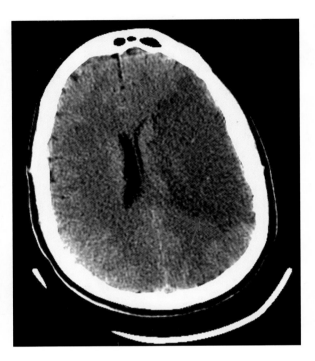

42. **The answer is A: Oral administration of 325 mg aspirin.** The CT scan shows a completed infarct (straight arrows) of the left MCA territory. The thrombus is identified within the left MCA on the left image as the *dense MCA sign* (curved arrow). Current AHA/ASA recommendations published in 2007 recommend the oral administration of aspirin (initial dose is 325 mg) within 24-48 hours after stroke onset for treatment of most patients.

B. Selected patients would have to present within 6 hours of the onset of symptoms for emergent administration of intraarterial rtPA to be a consideration.

C. Emergent CT perfusion study is indicated when the patient presents in a time frame where neurointerventional thrombolysis or thrombectomy is a consideration. It provides the interventionalist with additional information about the size of the core infarct and the amount of potentially salvageable tissue within the affected vascular territory.

D. Emergent neuroangiography with thrombectomy may be an option for selected patients who present in less than 6 hours from the onset of symptoms.

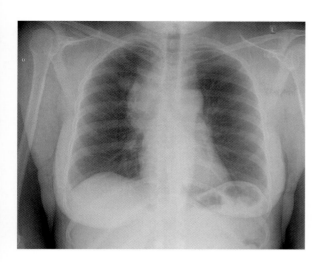

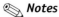

43. A 50-year-old woman visits her primary care physician complaining of gradually increasing shortness of breath. She has a history of mild asthma and has smoked one pack of cigarettes a day for 10 years. On physical examination, she has facial swelling, distended neck veins, and prominent superficial veins on her chest wall. A chest x-ray is obtained for further evaluation.

What is the most likely diagnosis?

A. Asthma exacerbation
B. Lung cancer
C. Lymphoma
D. TB
E. Pulmonary embolism

Superior Vena Cava (SVC Syndrome)

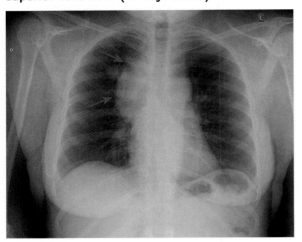

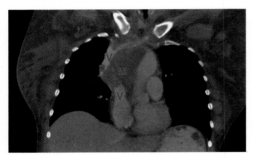

malignancy. A chest CT study (bottom) confirms a bulky mediastinal mass (M) causing nearly complete obstruction of the SVC (V).

SVCS is caused by malignant obstruction of the SVC in about 80% of cases. Among malignant cases, about 85% are caused by bronchogenic carcinoma, with about 15% caused by non-Hodgkin lymphoma. Prognosis for SVCS from bronchogenic carcinoma is poor, with 90% mortality at 30 months, despite treatment with radiation and chemotherapy. Without radiation, most are dead within a month. Endovascular stent placement to open the SVC is helpful for palliation.

A. Although the patient has a history of asthma, her symptoms and chest x-ray findings are more typical of SVCS from a large mediastinal mass. The expected chest x-ray findings in a patient with asthma exacerbation would be pulmonary hyperinflation, sometimes with patchy areas of atelectasis if there is mucous plugging from secretions.
C. Lymphoma can cause obstruction of the SVC but less often than bronchogenic carcinoma.
D. TB and other granulomatous diseases, such as histoplasmosis, can cause mediastinal adenopathy and mediastinal fibrosis, which may result in SVCS. These etiologies of SVCS are more common in developing countries where TB is more prevalent. In the United States, bronchogenic carcinoma is a far more likely cause.
E. Pulmonary embolism may cause dyspnea, and some patients have recognizable pulmonary artery enlargement on the chest x-ray. However, this patient has a bulky mediastinal mass and no pulmonary arterial enlargement.

43. **The answer is B: Lung cancer.** The patient's symptoms of dyspnea with physical signs of facial edema, distended neck veins, and prominent collateral veins on the chest wall are characteristic of superior vena cava syndrome (SVCS), an obstruction of the SVC most commonly caused by lung cancer.

The chest x-ray (top) confirms a large mediastinal mass, predominantly right-sided, in the region of the SVC (arrows), and highly suspicious for

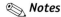

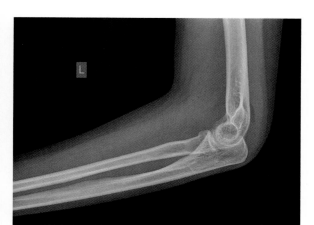

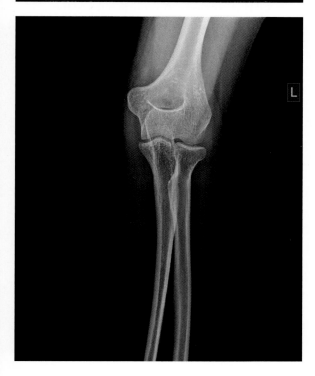

44. A 32-year-old woman presents to her primary care physician with pain in her left elbow after falling while roller-blading 2 days ago and bracing her fall with her outstretched left arm. On physical exam, there is swelling and diffuse tenderness involving the left elbow. Radiographs are obtained. Which of the following statements is true?

A. The anterior fat pad is elevated.
B. The posterior fat pad is not displaced.
C. There is no joint effusion.
D. There is no fracture.
E. A supracondylar fracture is highly likely.

Elbow Joint Effusion and Radial Head Fracture

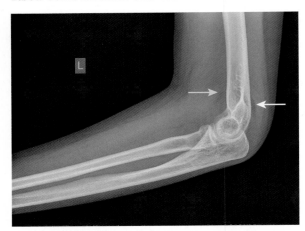

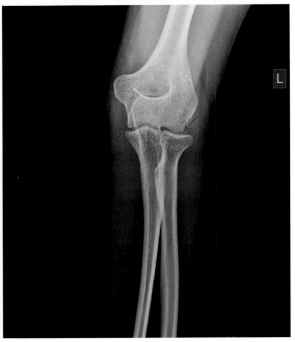

44. **The answer is A: The anterior fat pad is elevated.** The patient presents with a FOOSH-type injury. In the adult population, a FOOSH mechanism can result in injury at the wrist, elbow, or shoulder. Based on the lateral radiograph shown, there is displacement of both the anterior (yellow arrow) and posterior (white arrow) fat pads, from the anterior and posterior olecranon fossae, respectively, indicating the presence of a joint effusion.

In young adults, the most common elbow fracture involves the radial head (50%), is usually nondisplaced (< 2 mm), and results from low-energy axial loading in a FOOSH mechanism. It is normal to see the oblique anterior fat pad on a lateral radiograph, but when elevated, producing the so-called sail sign, an effusion is present. It is never normal to see the posterior fat pad. A nondisplaced radial head fracture is often occult/subtle on radiographs; nevertheless, the presence of an effusion without other obvious fracture, dislocation, or other joint derangement highly suggests the presence of a radial head fracture. Treatment of a nondisplaced radial head fracture is usually limited to nonsteroidal antiinflammatory drugs and physical therapy, with early mobilization key to a good prognosis.

B. The fat pad is displaced as noted.
C. A joint effusion is present.
D. On the AP radiograph shown, though subtle, the vertical component of a radial head fracture (red arrow) can be seen in the midportion of the articular surface. Nevertheless, in the setting of trauma, a joint effusion indicates fracture until proven otherwise, and in adults a radial head fracture is most common.
E. In children, the most common elbow fracture is a supracondylar fracture.

Section IV
ANSWER KEYS

USMLE | CONSULT
STEPS ❶❷❸

About   Contributors   Free Trial   Purchase   Testimonials

Step 1

My USMLE Consult
Create a Test
Previous Tests
Resume Incomplete
Tests
Cumulative Results
Compare My Results to
Others
Results Over Time

TELL A FRIEND

▶ Share USMLE with a
friend!

Back to Previous Tests

Review Test
Jan 16, 2010 4:55 PM EST to Sep 8, 2011 10:34 AM EST

Test Results | **Review Test** | Incorrect Questions by Disciplines | Incorrect Questions by Organ Systems

Listed below are your questions. You can review the questions by clicking on the "Question" and the "High-yield Hit" links next to each question.

#	Correct	Disciplines	Organ Systems	Time	Review	%Correct[1]
1.	✓	Behavioral Science	General	40 sec.	Question	37%
2.	✓	Gross Anatomy	Gastrointestinal	28 sec.	Question	56%
3.	✓	Behavioral Science	General	12 sec.	Question	45%
4.	✕	Neuroscience	Nervous	14 sec.	Question	77%
5.	✓	Pharmacology/Therapeutics	Nervous	20 sec.	Question	47%
6.	✓	Gross Anatomy	Cardiovascular	300 sec.	Question	53%
7.	✓	Embryology	Nervous	11 sec.	Question	86%
8.	✕	Immunology	Hematopoietic/ Lymphoid	33 sec.	Question	39%
9.	✕	Histology	Reproductive	36 sec.	Question	51%
10.	✕	Biochemistry	Cardiovascular	11 sec.	Question	55%
11.	✕	Immunology	Hematopoietic/ Lymphoid	52 sec.	Question	46%
12.	✓	Neuroscience	Nervous	19 sec.	Question	77%
13.	✕	Pathology	General	32 sec.	Question	64%

Section I BOARD IMAGES

Question 1: E	Question 30: A	Question 59: E	Question 88: E
Question 2: E	Question 31: A	Question 60: E	Question 89: C
Question 3: B	Question 32: A	Question 61: C	Question 90: A
Question 4: E	Question 33: D	Question 62: E	Question 91: B
Question 5: A	Question 34: C	Question 63: B	Question 92: B
Question 6: A	Question 35: A	Question 64: D	Question 93: A
Question 7: D	Question 36: C	Question 65: D	Question 94: C
Question 8: B	Question 37: A	Question 66: C	Question 95: E
Question 9: A	Question 38: B	Question 67: A	Question 96: E
Question 10: F	Question 39: A	Question 68: D	Question 97: E
Question 11: F	Question 40: E	Question 69: D	Question 98: C
Question 12: A	Question 41: A	Question 70: A	Question 99: D
Question 13: D	Question 42: E	Question 71: D	Question 100: D
Question 14: D	Question 43: B	Question 72: A	Question 101: E
Question 15: C	Question 44: E	Question 73: B	Question 102: E
Question 16: D	Question 45: C	Question 74: D	Question 103: A
Question 17: B	Question 46: B	Question 75: C	Question 104: D
Question 18: E	Question 47: A	Question 76: D	Question 105: E
Question 19: D	Question 48: D	Question 77: C	Question 106: D
Question 20: E	Question 49: B	Question 78: F	Question 107: D
Question 21: B	Question 50: C	Question 79: B	Question 108: C
Question 22: B	Question 51: E	Question 80: B	Question 109: C
Question 23: E	Question 52: A	Question 81: C	Question 110: E
Question 24: B	Question 53: C	Question 82: B	Question 111: C
Question 25: E	Question 54: D	Question 83: B	Question 112: A
Question 26: E	Question 55: E	Question 84: E	Question 113: B
Question 27: E	Question 56: B	Question 85: B	Question 114: A
Question 28: C	Question 57: B	Question 86: B	
Question 29: D	Question 58: A	Question 87: A	

Section II CARDIOLOGY

Question 1: E	Question 6: B	Question 11: B	Question 16: C
Question 2: D	Question 7: E	Question 12: B	Question 17: B
Question 3: B	Question 8: A	Question 13: C	Question 18: D
Question 4: A	Question 9: A	Question 14: D	Question 19: E
Question 5: B	Question 10: D	Question 15: A	Question 20: D

Section III RADIOLOGY

Question 1: C	Question 12: C	Question 23: B	Question 34: C
Question 2: A	Question 13: B	Question 24: E	Question 35: E
Question 3: D	Question 14: A	Question 25: E	Question 36: D
Question 4: B	Question 15: D	Question 26: D	Question 37: C
Question 5: E	Question 16: B	Question 27: B	Question 38: D
Question 6: A	Question 17: C	Question 28: D	Question 39: C
Question 7: C	Question 18: C	Question 29: E	Question 40: C
Question 8: C	Question 19: D	Question 30: A	Question 41: E
Question 9: A	Question 20: C	Question 31: B	Question 42: A
Question 10: B	Question 21: C	Question 32: C	Question 43: B
Question 11: E	Question 22: D	Question 33: D	Question 44: A

Index